HELPING YOUR CHILD
BE WELL

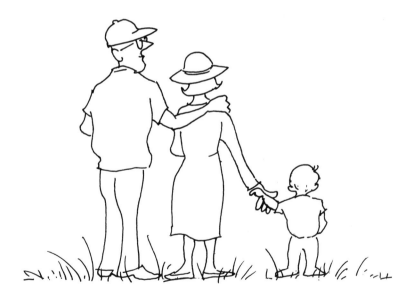

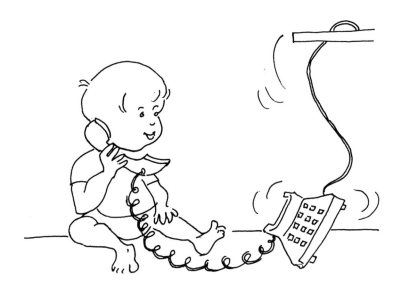

HELPING YOUR CHILD
BE WELL

A Pediatrician's 101 True Stories
and Vignettes About Childhood Diseases,
Prevention, Health, and Happiness

By

RAGHAVENDRA A. N. RAO, M.D.

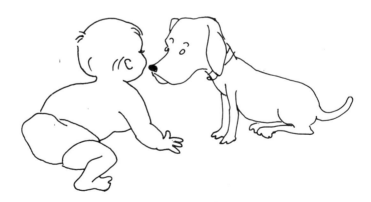

Published by:

ISP Publications
37-07 74th Street
Jackson Heights, NY 11372
info@isppublications.com
www.isppublications.com

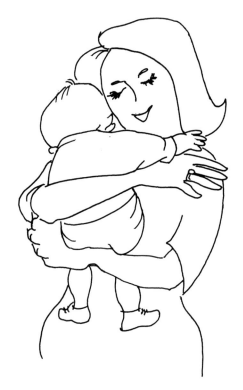

First Edition 2004

ISBN: 0-9749761-0-5

Cover, illustrations & book design by Gopi Gajwani
This book is printed on acid free paper.
The typefont used is Garamond

A hundred years from now
it will not matter
what my bank account was,
the sort of house I lived in, or
the kind of car I drove,
but the world may be different
because I was important
in the life of a child.

KATHY DAVIS

The glory of Medicine is that
it is constantly moving forward, that
there is always more to learn.

WILLIAM MAYO

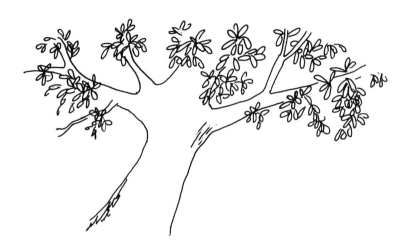

Dedicated to all the children who, over the years,
brightened my office with their smiles, and taught me
love, compassion, and humility.

In memory of my parents
Srinivasa Rao and Krishnamma

Acknowledgments

I thank ISP Publications for their suggestions and support, and Mrs. Shirley Hickman for her comments on several of the stories. Grateful acknowledgment is made to the *Porterville Recorder* in which many of the stories first appeared. Many thanks also go to my daughters, Geetha and Veena, and to my son-in-law, Raja, all of whom offered valuable suggestions and diligently checked each and every story in spite of their own busy schedules as doctors. Finally, I am indebted to Usha, my wife, for her patience and support; without her help, I would not have been able to write this book.

Contents

Prevention and Cure

Health and Nutrition

Drugs and the Innocent

Heredity and Genes

Wonders of Medicine

Evolution of Medicine

Medical Curiosity

Medical Detective

Against all Odds

Family Support and the Power of Prayer

Fun, Frolic, and Afterthoughts

Preface

Every child has a scary story to tell, but the stories that parents face are scarier. Weighed down with responsibility, they often do not know what to do. This is especially true with new parents, and with parents who are either very young or have come to parenthood late in life. One child develops a sore throat. Another runs a fever. In school, a classmate comes down with an infectious disease. What is a parent to do? When does one take care of a symptom at home, and when does one run to a doctor?

These are troublesome questions that every parent faces. Feelings of guilt come into play. "Am I delaying too long? What if something bad happens?" comes to a caring parent's mind. "Would I forgive myself then?"

"Should I really call the doctor at this hour?" another parent asks, as a child's fever rises and the clock's hands point to midnight. "Should we rush to the emergency room instead?" Bothersome, even frightening possibilities crowd the mind. What if? What if?

In my long years of practice I have learned that it is not just bodies that need to be treated. Minds must also be set at ease. This book attempts to set parental minds at ease, by showing how a pediatrician handles the many crises of childhood that come before him. I will address these questions, which I will call "bugs and drugs," from the point of view both of a pediatrician and a parent.

Let me stress, right away, the importance of prevention. The saying that "prevention is better than cure" is more than a proverb; it is a truism that we parents and doctors should apply in our personal and professional lives. Since the advent of antibiotics and antiviral agents, we know that most common infections can be tackled efficiently and swiftly but we also know that infections such as whooping cough, measles, chicken pox, hepatitis A and B, and certain meningeal infections are preventable by administering the proper vaccinations. Unfortunately, many parents and adolescents are unaware of this, or think they can beat the odds, or seek help too late. Because of this, more than 10 percent of infants and children in this country have not completed their immunizations. Your child should not be one of them. Many such children fall victim to diseases that can be transmitted from animals and contaminated foods. This is the "bug" problem.

Millions of adolescents and teenagers smoke, use and abuse drugs, and consume alcohol. They eat unhealthy foods. In my own practice, I have several teenagers weighing over 200 pounds. They have developed sedentary lifestyles that include long hours of watching television, playing video games, or surfing the internet. Because of these addictions, life-threatening diseases such as diabetes and high blood pressure are on the rise, and their complications are causing considerable morbidity. Further, innumerable problems like developmental delays, attention deficit disorders, and congenital malformations are noticed in children born to mothers who have abused drugs and alcohol. This is the "drug" problem.

Pregnancy and violence have become an astronomical problem among teenagers. Every year, 500,000 teenagers give birth in the United States. At the same time, gun usage to commit violent crimes has more than doubled since 1976. More teens die of violence than from a disease. Support, unconditional love, and hugs are missing in most families where violence prevails. I do advocate hugs as an essential element in family support. They may not cure an illness, but they certainly promote well-being. Hugs therefore are part of the solution.

In these pages I present problems as they occur in my pediatric practice, and offer solutions where solutions are possible, given the current state of medical science. Children make up 20 percent of this nation's population and 100 percent of our future. They are the architects of tomorrow's society and the foundation of its well-being. We need to face their issues now and try to resolve them to the best of our ability.

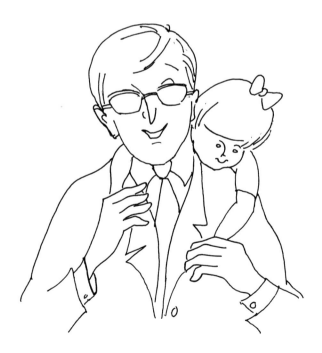

Introduction:
Protecting Your Unborn Child

In order to understand some of the diseases that affect children, we need to go to what happens in a would-be mother's womb. After conception, a fertilized egg divides rapidly. Eventually it will differentiate into 50 trillion cells to make a newborn baby!

At eight weeks, the fetus can hear the mother's heartbeat, rumblings of the intestines and the stomach, and her muffled voice. According to an Indian legend, a mythological Hindu king, soon after he was born, began chanting the god Vishnu's glories because, while still in the womb, he had heard a sage narrate them to his mother. Of course this is a myth, but we now have ample evidence that newborn babies can indeed recognize their mother's voice at birth.

At about 20 weeks, the baby starts to move and kick; any loud sound or sudden movement will make the baby react in this manner inside. Until the seventh month, there is a lot of space for the baby to even turn somersaults, sometimes getting entangled in the umbilical cord and miraculously coming out of it, a feat that Houdini would be proud of. It is dark in the womb and the warm and turbid amniotic fluid bathes the baby constantly, making the skin wrinkle.

Once the kidneys function, the baby voids freely into the amniotic fluid, now and then exhibiting strong sucking movements and swallowing mouthfuls of the urine-amniotic fluid mixture. Voiding, sucking, and moving around are complex functions and reflect the intricate nerve connections that are developing rapidly. Finally the baby settles in an upside-down yoga posture, ready to venture into the world at any moment.

While in the womb, the fetus is firmly attached to the uterus through a placenta, which can be compared to a parcel terminal, busily importing nutrients and oxygen, and exporting waste materials such as carbon dioxide and urea. Even though the placenta acts like a sieve and filters out most chemicals and germs before they reach the fetus, some bacteria and viruses can still pass through the barrier and access the rapidly dividing and growing cells, such as those of the brain, liver, and heart that are very vulnerable to damage.

To judge the potential for damage, we need only consider that the brain is growing at an awesome rate of 100,000 cells a minute! By the time the baby is born its brain has acquired 100 billion cells, all interconnected and ready to absorb information like a sponge. Any damage to these cells causes problems later, such as mental retardation, abnormal behaviors, and attention deficit disorders. Many childhood diseases are now identified by whatever agent caused an injury to the fetus in the womb; hence we get such names as "Thalidomide baby" and "congenital rubella syndrome".

Infections and their effects

If viruses and bacteria cross the placenta to infect the fetus, especially in the first 12 weeks of pregnancy, the damage to the rapidly multiplying cells can result in devastating congenital malformations, if not death. When a pregnant mother gets an infection called rubella, she herself hardly suffers physically. She may have a little cold, cough, and a sore throat, with a mild fever and a fine red rash all over her skin. The disease is named after the rash, as a reddish tinge in Latin is called *rubellus*. However, the rubella virus can easily cross the placental barrier and infect the fetus. If this happens, especially in the first eight weeks of pregnancy, spontaneous abortion, stillbirth, or major birth defects of the heart, eyes, or nervous system can occur; the infant may also be born with mental retardation, liver failure, deafness, and cataracts. This disease is called congenital rubella syndrome.

Even though rare now, I have seen several children with congenital rubella syndrome with all the concomitant problems that I have mentioned. Recently I took care of Heather, an 11- year-old girl with mental retardation, flat feet, eye defect, and malformation of her pulmonary artery. She had an uncontrollable behavior of rocking back and forth and an obsessive touching of her ears, tongue, and chin with her fingers. She lives with her foster mother; no one knows where her real mother is. I also know a couple of blind adults with mental retardation and severe behavioral problems who are affected by the syndrome; they live in a nearby state facility and need 24-hour total care. The sad part of it is, that this eventuality is totally preventable nowadays.

A vaccine to prevent the disease was introduced in 1969. Between 1964 and 1965 we had a pandemic of rubella; in just those two years, twelve million people were infected with the disease and 20,000 infants were born with congenital rubella syndrome. After the vaccine was introduced, fewer than 200 people are affected with rubella annually, and fewer than 12 newborns are seen with congenital rubella syndrome. A remarkable achievement in preventive medicine!

Other infections, such as toxoplasmosis, chicken pox, and syphilis can cause similar problems. High fever due to any infection in early pregnancy may precipitate abortion or lead to spinal defects and other malformations. A vaccine that is now available is 85 to 95 percent effective in preventing the chicken pox infection, and should be given routinely to children.

Yet, some mothers are reluctant to get their children immunized. Some believe that natural immunity offers better protection and hence children do not need vaccinations. Some are afraid of the potential complications of vaccination; others believe herbs will protect their children against diseases. Many teenagers and young adults, with an "It's not going to happen to me" attitude, ignore medical advice and appointments. Unfortunately, their children suffer just like Heather.

Medication and its side effects

Sadly, not all medication works the way it is supposed to. In 1957, a German pharmaceutical company introduced a sedative called Thalidomide. Many pregnant women took this medication to combat sleeplessness. Later, hundreds of babies were born without arms, legs, toes, or fingers, and had other congenital malformations. These infants were known as "Thalidomide babies", and the medication was immediately withdrawn from the market.

Since then, we have become aware that many medications can cause severe problems to the baby, especially if they are taken during the early stages of pregnancy. For example, phenytoin, a medicine used to treat seizures, can cause multiple problems, such as congenital malformations, intrauterine growth retardation, bleeding, and cancerous tumors called neuroblastomas. Tetracycline, an antibiotic, causes limb malformation, defective bone growth, cataracts, and tooth problems.

Generally speaking, major abnormalities develop if the fetus is exposed to the medication in the first few weeks of pregnancy. After the third month, minor defects and physiologic abnormalities, such as enzyme defects, are more likely. The ill effects of a medication taken during pregnancy may not become evident in the child till later on in life. Adolescent girls have developed adenocarcinoma, a cancer of the vagina. We know now that these unfortunate teenagers were exposed to a hormone called Diethylstilbestrol, which their mothers took during pregnancy. Similarly, intrauterine exposure of the fetus to phenytoin and alcohol may later result in childhood tumors.

It is true that pregnant women need supplemental vitamins like folic acid that prevent neural tube defects. Many think that vitamins are innocuous and swallow mega-doses with no hesitation. However, huge doses of vitamins are harmful to the mother and the fetus. Vitamin D, if consumed in excess, can result in increased level of calcium that is potentially harmful, and a narrowing of the major blood vessel in the newborn, the aorta.

Perhaps we are not spending enough time with the target population to educate and inform them about these complications. It is worrisome to note that 90 percent of pregnant women have taken at least one medication, and an average pregnant woman has consumed four medicines other than iron or vitamins. Incredibly, 4 percent of women in pregnancy have used ten or more medications. In addition, many are exposed to pesticides, hair sprays, and other chemicals whose effects on the fetus are unknown.

So I would urge all women to beware: no medication should be given to a pregnant mother, unless it is thought to be absolutely necessary.

Drugs and their effects

It is hard to believe but true that many eighth graders use drugs. About 9 percent of eighth graders, 18 percent of 10th graders, and 24.6 percent of 12th graders smoke on a daily basis. In a

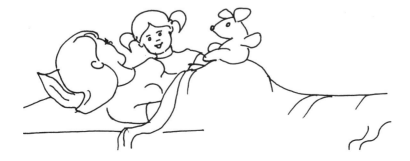

national study in 1999, 51 percent of high school seniors had consumed alcoholic drinks, 34.6 percent had smoked cigarettes, 23.1 percent had used marijuana, 2.7 percent had abused LSD, and 2.6 percent had tried cocaine in the 30 days preceding the survey. Nearly 12 percent of high school seniors have tried Ecstasy at least once. Scary statistics!

Alcohol, cigarettes, marijuana, and Ecstasy are the four most commonly used drugs. Usually their usage leads to the use of other, more harmful drugs. Teenagers who smoke cigarettes, drink alcohol, or use marijuana at 14 or15 years of age are likely to abuse illicit drugs later on in their lives.

Cultural and societal norms, peer pressure, and adult role models influence a teenager's use of drugs. Drug abuse on the other hand is related to biological and psychological factors. For example, a tendency to alcohol addiction is genetically inherited.

A teenager uses drugs because he is unhappy with his life and the drugs give him an immediate, intense pleasure; what the teen cannot realize is that a satisfying relationship between a parent and a child brings long-lasting happiness. When such a satisfying relationship and bonding is wanting, the teen searches for pleasure elsewhere. This causes further alienation, and a break-down of family love and relationships.

Sometimes we give our children a confusing message. Drinking at parties is an accepted social norm, as is popping open a champagne bottle on New Year's Eve with lots of laughter and clapping of hands. Children, especially those under the age of six, keenly watch what their parents do. Their rapidly growing brain cells get wired to acknowledge that drinking is enjoyable and desirable. And they do so later on. Some, due to genetic and psychological reasons, become addicted to alcohol.

Why am I worried about drugs? Drugs contribute to the three leading causes of death among adolescents, namely, accidents, homicide, and suicide. Multiple organs are damaged leading to heart attacks, liver failure, and brain damage. Adolescents who abuse drugs do not develop the educational and social skills needed to handle the complex problems of the world, and rarely do they grow into independent, successful, and responsible adults.

Sadly, drugs cause damage to the child in the womb too. Alcohol consumption by the mother can cause heart and nervous system abnormalities, limb defects, intrauterine growth retardation, attention deficit disorder, and autism. Cocaine causes the child to have a small head, growth retardation, blood vessel malformations, and behavioral problems. Women who smoke are ten times more likely to have miscarriages than nonsmokers, and their children tend to have low birth weight. I have taken care of a few children with behavioral problems, pulmonary stenosis, and attention deficit disorders who were born to addicted mothers. It seems so unfair that a child should suffer because of a mother's nonchalant indulgence in drugs.

Violence and its effects

The majority of adolescents and adults are law abiding and peaceful. But violence rears its ugly head frequently enough to be classified as a national epidemic.

Children are initially exposed to violence at home. About 1.8 million women in this country are regularly beaten by their spouses each year; wives are battered in 16 percent of families. That is roughly one in every six married women! Family violence happens usually in the child-rearing years, and it is estimated that 3.3 million children witness domestic violence every year in the United States. When I was training in hematology, I knew a child whose father had shot her mother in her presence.

Children often see violence in the form of sexual assault. In Los Angeles County, the sheriff's sexual assault investigators estimate that a child is present at 50 percent of rapes that occur at home, and that about 10 percent of children witness the rape. In addition, adults subject many children to physical, verbal, and psychological abuse. One child out of 25 is abused and 2000 children die annually as a result of such abuse in this country.

Children are also exposed to community violence quite frequently. A study of first and second grade children in Washington, DC, showed that 45 percent of them had seen a mugging, 47 percent a shooting, and 31 percent a stabbing, while 39 percent had seen a dead body. About 10 percent of children who attended the pediatric clinic in Boston City hospital had witnessed a shooting or a stabbing before the age of six. In New Orleans, one third of school children have witnessed a severe violent act. Obviously, children are exposed to more violent acts in urban and some inner city areas.

Another source of violence is television. Naturally occurring disasters, serial killings, bombings, and sniper attacks are televised relentlessly even in prime hours. An average child between two and five years of age watches 20 to 30 hours of television a week, many of which are filled with violent scenes. Many video games are very violent, and the level of violence increases as the game progresses.

What are the effects of violence on children?

Some children erroneously conclude that violence is one way to solve problems or reduce tension. Recent school shootings give ample credence to such beliefs. Girls who are raised in families with domestic violence are more likely to become victims of battering themselves. Boys growing up in violent families are likely to batter their wives as adults. Recent studies by PET scans have shown that structural changes occur in the brains of children exposed to violence early in life. As a result, later on, children and adolescents exhibit behavior problems, repression, violence, and suicidal tendencies. In addition they may suffer with various health problems, such as vague stomachaches, stress, eating disorders, regression, and sleeplessness.

Children crave quality time

Hitherto, I have been painting a dismal picture of the problems that children and adolescents face. The majority of children grow up normal, well behaved, and responsible. They are loved by their parents and in turn return the love and trust. However, the problems I have mentioned do exist, and we have to tackle them to give our children a healthier life, both in body and mind.

In these days of managed health care, there is a tendency for physicians to spend less and less time with children and their families. Parents too, I observe, spend less time with their children for various reasons. Often parents need to work to make ends meet. The same trend is present in single-parent families. Children are spending their time more often either in a daycare center, with a baby sitter, or at home alone glued to a television or video game.

I have known families where both parents work from dawn to dusk. They are well off, have a luxurious house, a pool, and nice cars, but their children hardly see them. The children don't want their parent's profession. In other words, they are craving for more attention and quality time from their parents.

Here, I would like to share my thoughts on importance of the family and sound communication in raising children and its value in healing diseases. I will briefly touch on the importance of building a strong support system both within the family and in the community to better serve the needs of children.

Bedtime stories shaped values

I grew up in a sizable family with four brothers and three sisters. My father, Srinivasa Rao, was a teacher. He was a very good storyteller. Usually at bedtime, either he or an aunt would assemble all of us and tell us stories, which always had moral values, such as "If you harm others, you will be harmed at the end", "Riches are transient, Knowledge is permanent", and so on.

At a young age I was exposed to two great Indian epics, the Ramayana and Mahabharata, which apart from being wonderful classics, also provided readers and hearers with gems of moral values, meaningful aphorisms, and everlasting truths. I did not understand much at that time, but now I realize their profound influence on me. Moreover, my father used to bring a lot of books from the school library and encouraged me to read. All these activities molded my character and made me what I am now.

My father had a few simple rules. After play, we had to wash well—we played in the village streets that were full of dust—and had to study at least for an hour. We sat around a hurricane lamp and read aloud, raising a cacophony. Studies were very important in his view. When I bragged, he would cut me off, saying, "A man who talks will be talking for ever; a man of action will do the job." Just like the rules taught in kindergarten nowadays, he instilled certain rules and values in me early in my life.

My mother was a homemaker, but she had another role to play. When my father got upset with us for some reason or other, my mother was there on our side to give full support. Thus a balance was maintained in our family, which I think is essential for children's normal growth and development.

Growing up in a big family, I had my share of squabbles. But I learned to give and take, picked up the art of negotiation, and developed the ability to adjust. When I fell ill, in addition to my parents, my sisters and brothers hovered near me looking after my comfort. I was a king, for a while. I felt what love was and learned to share it with others.

In big families, tension is diffused as other family members offer physical and psychological support. When my beloved aunt died, there was much sorrow in our family, but by mutual support and love we got over the depression within a short time.

Such large and extended families were common in the early part of the twentieth century, even in this country, but family size has been shrinking slowly. In the past 40 years, the average family size has decreased from 3.67 to 3.18 members. Moreover, the number of married-couple families has also declined. When both parents work they have less time to spend with their children. All this generally translates into poor communication, inability to resolve conflicts, and insufficient emotional support.

As a parent and a pediatrician, I believe that one needs to pay heed to certain important factors, to enable children to grow and develop in positive, healthy ways both in body and mind.

Communication from an early age

Mrs. Gerber brings her six-year old daughter, Amber, to my office. When she was pregnant, she patiently read stories and sang nursery rhymes to the baby in her womb. Mrs. Gerber told me that Amber kicked when she sang lullabies. She was sure that Amber had heard her voice. Later, during office visits, Mrs. Gerber would explain softly to Amber that she would receive some shots. It would hurt, but the vaccines were for her good. She would assure Amber that her pain would subside with Tylenol.

Mrs. Gerber often brought a book and read it to Amber while waiting in the office. As Amber grew up she was so well behaved that I could explain things to her easily without any protest from her. All this, I believe, was because Mrs. Gerber took time to explain and communicate with her child early on.

I have two daughters, Geetha and Veena. When they were young, our family of four would make it a point to eat dinner together; we talked about school, the day's incidents, and other matters, problems, and frustrations. We openly expressed ourselves, and solutions were discussed. Like a scientist, I would analyze the problems and offer an answer, often dry and unpalatable. On the other hand, my wife Usha would add a human touch to my scientific analysis that the girls would readily agree and follow. This worked well for our family.

I did not realize it then, but now it is obvious that those moments molded my daughters' future. I used to narrate interesting stories about children whom I treated, like those in my book. I sowed the seed of medical curiosity in them. Both grew up to become physicians, Geetha a geriatric specialist and Veena an internist. Geetha jokes with me, "Dad, together we can handle problems from the cradle to the grave!"

Communication is an art. With children, commands and preaching will usually fall on deaf ears. Negative instructions, such as "do what I say" or "boys of your age should know better" are detrimental and counter productive. Instead, replace them with positive comments like, "you did a good job fixing your room" or "I'm proud of you. You have finished your home work so soon."

Long ago, I took care of Monica, a teenager who usually was accompanied by her mother. I never saw Monica's father. The mother had a limp and carried a cane for support. She had a huge list of complaints against Monica. This family specialized in constant arguments even at my office. When the mother would tell me something, Monica would say the exact opposite.

Every now and then the mother would tap Monica with her cane. "Stop it mom, it's so embarrassing," Monica would protest. I did my best to counsel them and refer them to a psychologist. Monica's mother never stopped nagging. Eventually, Monica dated a teenager against her mother's will and became pregnant. This family is a good example of poor communication.

In families where children are constantly criticized, nagged, blamed, threatened, and punished, this is very detrimental to their development. On the other hand, they thrive when we treat them with love, provide them with support, trust and encourage them, and teach them the art of negotiation and good communication.

Communication also involves setting a good example as well as making a few sacrifices. A parent who smokes cannot expect his children not to smoke. The same applies to alcohol or drug abuse. Being a good role model is of paramount importance while bringing up children.

In my office, communication plays a vital role. Greeting the parents and calling a child by his or her first name makes them happy and comfortable. I engage small children, three or four years old, in small talk to facilitate examination. While examining the mouth I may say, "Gee, Sara, you have a big mouth. A cheeseburger would easily fit here!" Children are happy about eating food and they relax at my comments, or I may say, "Sara, who has more teeth, you or a shark?" Children are self-centered and invariably say, "Me!" which elicits laughter from the parents. In older children I break the ice by talking about sports or about an activity they are interested in, such as a youth club or band.

While taking the child's medical history I tend to be patient and unhurried. I use simple language devoid of medical jargon, and allow the parents to absorb and ask questions. Treatment plans for certain diseases, such as diabetes and asthma, are complicated. I go over them a couple of times to make sure that the parents or adolescents have understood the details. Sometimes I draw pictures that save time and clarify the issue.

Just like the "Kodak Moment", there is always a "Teaching Moment" in my practice. It can happen any time to educate a teenager or a parent. The talk is directed at the child's or family's specific needs. I usually keep my talk less than a minute unless parents ask questions.

Reading books aloud, taking family trips to a book store or library, working at hobbies with children, sharing household chores with them at every opportunity, are all different ways of communication. This is how you can express your love, praise, respect, and approval to your child.

An important aspect of communication is listening to your children. Take time to listen to them by blocking out distractions. Put yourself in your child's shoes. Maintain eye contact. Nod your head or say words of approval to indicate that you are paying attention.

When a family communicates effectively, they understand each other and learn each other's needs. Your love and care are the connections between you and your child. This will protect your child from going astray in these days of sleek advertisements about smoking, alcohol and sex. The skills your children learn now will help them to build confidence, face life and understand society.

Building community partnerships

Even though the onus of raising a child falls mainly on parents, the community also needs to share that responsibility. Friends, church, physician, school, police, media and other organizations should come together to help children develop strength both in body and mind.

In Porterville, a small town of 40,000 people, we have quite a few organizations that are fine-tuned to help families. I am a member of an organization called "Safe from the Start", which targets children from birth up to five years of age—a period of rapid brain growth—to prevent abuse and neglect and to educate parents about the ill effects of abuse.

Also, I participate in another organization, "Porterville Area Wellness Services," that promotes the idea that health care is a partnership among children, families, health personnel, and the community. We provide the necessary phone numbers for available resources and health information. We also provide limited monetary help.

I believe it is of paramount importance that we build a partnership with adolescents and parents, educating them in the areas of drug abuse, teenage pregnancy, and violence prevention. We are pouring money into building more and more prisons instead of supporting programs that keep people out of prison. We should have an accessible health care system to provide for early detection, prevention and treatment of conditions that lead to violence, teen pregnancy and drug abuse. There is a dearth of mental health care facilities for children and adolescents and money spent now in this area will go a long way in preventing child neglect and abuse in the next generation.

In a recent meeting we came up with a few interesting suggestions. They are:

- Lower fences in our backyards for better communication with neighbors.
- Institute home visit programs for high risk families at least once a week to educate them about basic health care.
- Build neighborhood communities and educate them through block-parties.
- Pair a teen mother with an experienced mother for guidance.

All of these are very welcome ideas.

Once a week, I visit local elementary schools to teach sixth grade students. I talk to them about the ill effects of tobacco and the dangers of alcohol and drug abuse. I use attractive, colorful slides to aid in my talk, which are devoid of any medical jargon. The school district has provided me several educational videos—a good example of partnership—that I play during my talk. More-

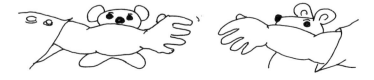

over, students in an elementary school have made a video of my rap song about the ill effects of tobacco. ("Listen to me, Don't be a fool!" from the story, "How Much Of Your Life Do You Want To Lose?") I play the video after the talk and the students like it very much. Involving children in the educational process is highly effective.

Healing power of prayer

I have treated many children and adolescents with cancer. They and their families constantly live with the fear of death. Even when they are free of cancer, they dread every laboratory test as it may show a relapse of the disease. They are tortured by anxiety, depression and suicidal thoughts and spend sleepless nights, stressed out.

One of my professors, Dr. Robinson, once told me about a five-year-old girl who was terminally ill in the hospital with cancer. One evening, she insisted on seeing her mother, who was at home. The on-call physician phoned the child's mother to come immediately to the hospital. The little girl hugged her mother and said that she had heard the bells ringing in heaven, summoning her. She died in a few moments. I believe that this little girl decided to quit fighting. Once the mind gave up, the body stopped functioning.

We are beginning to understand the awesome power of the mind over the body. People who habitually suppress their anger have higher incidence of hypertension. People of Type A personality—impatient, aggressive, and hostile— are prone for coronary heart disease, and those with hostility are most susceptible of all. People who are socially isolated, with feelings of hopelessness and loss of control, die prematurely.

To combat the stress and promote healing, people over the millennia have found solace in prayer and meditation. Coming from India, I strongly believe in the healing power of prayer. Here too, 82 percent of Americans believe in the healing quality of personal prayer. I advise prayer, attending Church services, and breathing exercises to alleviate fear, anxiety, and stress in children and their families. Sometimes I pray for a child's quick recovery.

Prayer has helped several of my patients. Brenda, a teenager with lymph node cancer benefited from it. Richard, who had a fear of tornadoes, came out of it because of his and the family's belief in God. Prayer helped parents of Dennis who died from leukemia at the tender age of two years.

Nowadays medical centers have special clinics staffed by qualified personnel knowledgeable in the techniques of stress reduction. They teach how to control breathing. Focusing on breath is very calming and an essential part of meditation. Many hospitals have chapels for meditation and prayer. Our local hospital has a small prayer room and a chaplain for religious services.

The true stories I present here are those of children who have come to my office with various problems, and the solutions to the problems. The children have taught me love, compassion, humility, and a sense of humor. I am indebted to them. I have changed the names of the children and parents to protect their privacy.

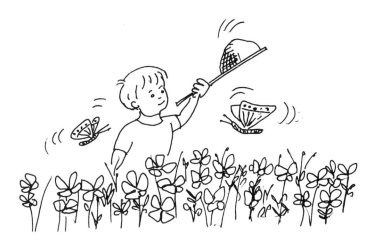

Croon a Tune!

Mrs. Gerber crooned a soothing tune. Hugging her two-month-old infant and looking into the baby's eyes, she said softly, "You see, Amber, Dr. Rao will give you three shots today for your own good. These shots will protect you against bad diseases. You don't need those bad things, do you?" She opened the Tylenol bottle and carefully measured 0.4 ml of the drops. Gently she put the drops in Amber's mouth. She picked Amber up, kissed her, and sweet-talked, "Amber, my baby, these shots hurt but only for a short time. I gave you Tylenol so the shots won't hurt you. When we go home we'll have a warm bath and you'll feel better. You'll sleep good. OK?"

I asked her, "Mrs. Gerber, do you talk to your baby like this, always?"

"Yes," she replied, "I even sang lullabies when Amber was in my tummy. She kicked when I sang. I think she knew I was singing."

A few years ago I would have been skeptical about such talk. Now I feel that there is some truth to these claims. This is because our understanding of early development of the brain has increased due to groundbreaking research in the past five years using PET scans and other imaging techniques.

At birth an infant has 100 billion nerve cells called neurons. Each neuron can make up to 15,000 connections, called synapses, with other neurons. These connections, like wiring, facilitate the passage of billions of signals from one part of the brain to another. Now we know that the majority of the connections develop during the first three years of life. The more the child is stimulated, the more connections develop and the more the child learns. By repeated stimulation some connections are reinforced and become permanent. This helps develop memory and knowledge. If not enough stimulation is provided, as in child deprivation or neglect, not enough connections are made. Moreover, some of the connections wither away, reducing the child's capacity to learn.

Tender loving care and constant interaction early in life have a long-lasting effect on a child's ability to learn and develop emotionally. New studies show that babies who receive warm care with positive stimulation in the first year of life are able to better handle stress later in life. Negative experiences or the absence of proper stimulation at critical periods will likely have serious long-term effects.

Mrs. Gerber has the right idea. So, play "Patty Cake" with your daughter. Read a book to your son. Pick up your newborn from the crib and croon a tune!

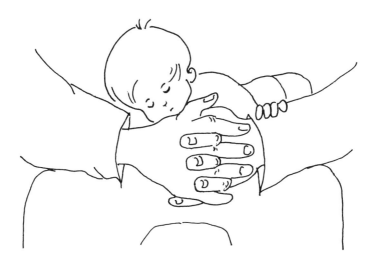

Newborn Screening —
A Boon to Infants

*T*erri, a pretty three-year-old girl, was brought to my office for a sore throat. As I examined her, I chatted with her mother. Terri had been born full term and was active and alert at birth. At the time of her discharge from the hospital, her doctor had requested a routine blood checkup called "Newborn Screen"; he was surprised when a laboratory test showed her total thyroxine (T4) was very low. Immediately, he requested several more tests to gauge Terri's thyroid functions.

The results had been startling. Because Terri's total thyroxine was so very low, her body was trying to prod the thyroid gland by secreting increased amounts of a thyroid stimulating hormone (TSH). Terri's TSH level was sky high. What was happening to the baby?

Terri was born with a condition called congenital hypothyroidism, which occurs in 1 in 4,000 births. Sometimes one finds a family history of hypothyroidism or goiter, but Terri's family had none. Congenital hypothyroidism is due to a developmental defect in the thyroid gland that causes it to secrete less of a hormone called thyroxine, which is needed for normal growth and development in children. An absence of this hormone from birth causes jaundice, constipation, and excess weight. Feeding difficulties, sluggishness, sleepiness, and breathing problems are often noted. A hypothyroid infant may have a protuberant abdomen, an umbilical hernia, and a low temperature. Later, anemia and heart failure may develop.

As the weeks go by, the child's muscles become weak and the skin becomes dry. The voice turns hoarse. Then growth is stunted, and the child develops mental retardation. Hence it is imperative to diagnose congenital hypothyroidism early and treat it effectively.

I have seen children who were diagnosed very late with hypothyroidism who have developmental delays; this happened because there were no newborn screening programs in those days. Thanks to such programs, we are now diagnosing several diseases such as phenylketonuria and hemoglobin disorders quite early, and thus preventing catastrophic consequences.

Terri was started on levothyroxine to replace the absent hormone, and she needed more thyroxine as she grew. Her thyroxine levels were periodically checked and the dosage of the medicine was adjusted. Terri is now growing well, just like any other child her age.

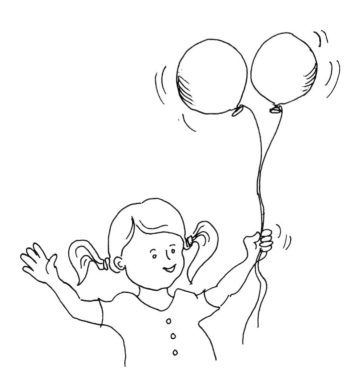

Does Breast-Feeding Improve IQ?

"What formula are you giving Angelica?" I asked Mrs. Gonzalez during a routine visit. Angelica was a cute one-year-old girl beginning to walk.

"I'm still breast-feeding," Mrs. Gonzalez replied hesitantly.

"Don't be embarrassed," I said. "You are not doing anything wrong. In many countries, mothers breast-feed for longer periods than is done here. Breast-milk is the best milk. Angelica is very cute and I bet she will be a very smart girl."

Mrs. Gonzalez took my last sentence as a compliment to her child, but what I said is very true: breast-feeding improves IQ.

Breast-feeding has many assets in addition to providing psychological benefits and bonding between mother and infant. Nursing infants have fewer allergies, asthma attacks, and eczema, which are frequently seen in formula-fed infants. Colic is uncommon.

Since many antibodies from the mother are present in breast-milk, the infant is protected against viral infections such as mumps, influenza, and rotavirus diarrhea. Children who are breast-fed also have fewer ear infections. A protein called lactoferrin in breast milk inhibits the growth of E. Coli, a deadly bacterium. Perhaps knowing this antibacterial and antiviral property, villagers in India treat eye infections by putting a few drops of fresh breast milk into the eyes of the affected person, which often clears the infection. A mother once told me that they do the same kind of treatment in Mexico.

Besides the above benefits, would you believe that breast-feeding actually increases a child's IQ? Full-term infants who were exclusively breast-fed for at least six months scored three points higher on their IQ tests at five years of age, when compared to infants who consumed formula or solid foods, or were breast-fed for a short period.

What about term infants born small? They are called 'small for gestational age' infants (SGA). A recent study in Norway and Sweden showed that SGA infants who were exclusively breast-fed during the first six months showed better overall cognitive development. Researchers evaluated these children at 3, 6, 9, and 13 months of age and again when they were 5 years old. They found that at 5 years of age, SGA children who were exclusively breast-fed at least for the first six months of life scored 11 points higher in IQ tests than those who were breast-fed for 12 weeks or less, or those who were given formula.

In the United States slightly more than 50 percent of mothers breast-feed. According to the 3rd National Health and Nutrition Examination Survey, only 21 percent of infants are exclusively breast-fed at the age of 4 months. By 6 months of age this number drops to 16 percent. Mothers, take notice. If you want smarter children, then breast-feed.

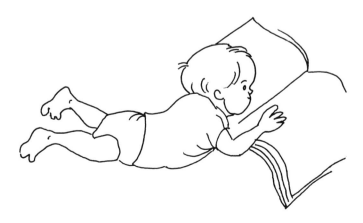

Please Look Into My Eyes, and Talk!

On a recent Halloween evening, a few goblins, witches, and cute princesses knocked at my door, less of them though than in previous years. When a big, bad witch gazed at me, I cringed involuntarily. When a princess looked at me, I was happy. In my office too, when I talk to children, some look at me and reply. Some look at the ceiling or the wallpaper, turn their faces away from me, or don't respond at all. It feels easy to talk with someone when face-to-face and eye-to-eye contact is made. It seems that an attractive person looks more attractive when he or she makes direct eye contact with the other person. Is there any scientific basis for these observations?

Yes, say the scientists. Recently, Kampe and others at the Institute of Cognitive Neuroscience in London have performed several elegant experiments. Sixteen volunteers, eight women and eight men, were shown color images of 40 different faces belonging to both sexes. These facial images had their eyes directed either at or away from the volunteer subject. When a volunteer was looking at the pictures, a functional magnetic resonance imaging (fMRI) study was done on the person's brain to document the areas of stimulation. It was found that an area called the ventral striatum of the brain was being stimulated during the sessions. After the fMRIs were taken, the volunteers were asked to rate from 1 to 10 the attractiveness of the facial images that they had seen, and the ratings were statistically analyzed. The results are very interesting.

When the eyes in the facial images were looking directly at the volunteer, the brain activity at the ventral striatum increased and the scores for attractiveness were high. When the eyes in the same facial images were looking away from the observer, the brain activity decreased and the attractive scores were less. When a volunteer felt that a facial image was unattractive, his scoring numbers were lower when the eyes in the picture were looking directly at him. When the eyes in the same unattractive image looked away, the volunteer's brain activity increased indicating a favorable response.

These findings translate into happiness and more social interaction when we perceive someone as attractive and he or she makes direct eye contact with us. When that person looks away, not bothering to make eye contact, we feel unhappy and social activity is curtailed. By the same token, when an unattractive person—unattractiveness being a personal viewpoint—gazes at us, we feel uneasy, and when that person looks away we feel comfortable. Animals follow basic survival trends that help them get close together with their kind or to escape from the gaze of a predator. These instincts are still with us. No wonder I cringed when the witch gazed into my eyes, and I smiled when the princess looked at me.

Young lovers, take note. Making eye contact early with your loved ones will enhance the appeal of a pleasant face and win their love!

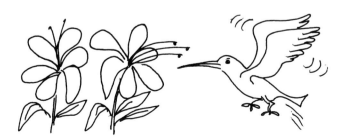

Animals, Asthma, and Children

Cathy and Lisa were sisters, six and eight years old respectively. They had moderate asthma and were on inhalant medications. Their asthma waxed and waned. Now and then they needed more medications to control their asthma. However, they were able to attend the school and participate in physical education.

"Many things precipitate or aggravate asthma," I told their mother. "Sometimes it can be exercise, or a surge in emotions. Or it can be animals, chemicals, cockroaches, rugs, dust mites, pollen, temperature changes, and tobacco smoke. In your case, it's your pet dog that's causing Cathy and Lisa to have those asthma attacks. You'll be better off giving it away."

"But, Dr. Rao, my children love the dog," Mrs. Lopez protested.

On a subsequent visit, I asked her whether she had been able to give the dog away. "No, Dr. Rao," she replied. "When I tried to, my kids got so upset that they started wheezing more."

A few years ago I would have been skeptical about such an answer. Nowadays, it is well known that asthma can be precipitated by emotional factors. When a child loves a pet, it is not possible to get rid of it without causing severe and sometimes devastating emotional problems. This, in turn, may aggravate asthma.

Children with asthma sometimes develop anxiety and depression. This is because their daily routines are disrupted due to asthma attacks, or by frequent visits to the doctor's office or admissions to a hospital. They need to carry medications at all times, even to camp. Parents get upset when they need to take time off from work to attend to a sick child, or when they spend sleepless nights administering aerosol medications. This compounds the anxiety in asthmatic children. Under such circumstances, the loss of a pet will heighten the anguish causing by a worsening of asthma.

Asthmatic children who have pets usually need more medication or more frequent use of medications. Even though it is a well-known fact that animals aggravate asthma, many children will not give away their pets. Studies have shown that only about 8 percent of children will get rid of their pets. Thus, a doctor sometimes has to make a difficult moral decision to allow an asthmatic child to have a pet, if giving it away would cause severe emotional problems. A happy child can be convinced to take medications regularly, resulting in a better management of asthma.

Our views are changing about the possible link between animals and allergies. Recent studies by Dr. Dennis Ownby of the Medical College of Georgia show that dogs and cats do not increase the risk of allergies in a child. In fact, if a child is raised in contact with animals early on in life, the risk of developing allergy is lessened. Scientists now feel that when a child is exposed to animals, its immune system is stimulated by the bacteria the animals carry. Thus, the child is better able to resist allergic diseases. Perhaps that is why children growing up in farms are less prone to allergies.

After a while, Cathy and Lisa knew that I was not pushing them to give away their pet.

"So, how many pets do you have now?" I casually asked one day.

"Four," Cathy replied. "We have two birds and two dogs."

Mrs. Lopez was smiling.

"What breed of dogs do you have?" I asked.

"One is just a dog; the other is a Dalmatian. We love them," beamed Cathy and Lisa happily.

"I know you love them. Just don't turn that one Dalmatian into one hundred and one Dalmatians, please!" I joked.

We all laughed. At that moment we forgot all about allergies and asthma.

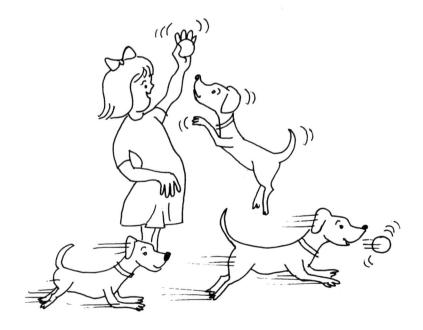

Flavor Favor

One day my wife Usha asked me, "Why are our children, Geetha and Veena, so finicky when it comes to eating? I've noticed that they relish chutney from their childhood. I like chutney too. Is this chutney-liking trait inherited?"

Usha like me is from India, the country that produced the Taj Mahal and tandoori chicken. I know what chutney is: a ground paste of lentils with various exotic spices, and it's delicious!

"I don't think there's any such thing as a chutney-liking trait," I said, smiling. "Since you like chutney, you have cooked it more often and offered it to our children, and that's probably how they developed a taste for it. For example, you know the taste for salty foods is acquired."

"It's true we eat chutney almost every day," she said, "but I offered our children other Indian foods, too. They still prefer chutney."

"I don't know why that is so," I said.

Recently I read an article about taste development in fetuses and newborns. It seems the taste buds develop around the 7th or 8th week of gestation; by 13 to 15 weeks, the taste buds resemble those of an adult. As the fetus develops, it starts sucking the amniotic fluid, which is full of chemicals like glucose, lactic acid, proteins, and urea. The urea comes from the urine that the fetus freely voids into the amniotic fluid. The developing fetus avidly sucks such a concoction—almost a liter a day—stimulating the taste buds. Taste is appreciated also through smell. The same amniotic fluid bathes and stimulates the olfactory apparatus situated in the upper part of the nose, thus enhancing the sensation of taste.

There are other chemicals found in the amniotic fluid, like traces of food items eaten by the mother. Amniotic fluid obtained from mothers who had consumed garlic 45 minutes before a routine amniocentesis, smelled like garlic. Spicy foods eaten by mothers impart their characteristic odors to the amniotic fluid. Needless to say the fetus tastes the foods *in utero* and is accustomed to some of the flavors even weeks before birth.

Soon after birth, infants can detect the odor of their mother's amniotic fluid. Day-old infants can recognize their mother's odors, especially those emanating from the volatile components of breast milk. All these indicate that an infant has a memory of taste and smell learned while in the womb. However, much still has to be learned in this field.

My children were exposed frequently to the taste and odor of chutney in the womb and while nursing, and liked it. Later, when chutney was offered, they recognized its flavor and enjoyed it.

Pregnant mothers beware! If you favor chips and coke, that is what your children will later like!

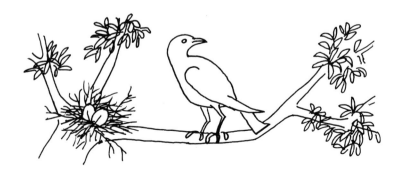

The Mark of Teenage Freedom

While walking in the Valley Plaza Mall, Mrs. Jones noticed a black mark on the ankle of her teenage daughter, Diane.

"Stop a second, Diane," said Mrs. Jones. "Something's sticking to your ankle."

"Nothing's sticking, mom, it's a tattoo."

Mrs. Jones was shocked; she could not believe that her intelligent daughter would do such a thing. Mrs. Jones had heard that tattoos could cause bacterial infections, Hepatitis B, and even AIDS when contaminated needles were used.

Diane got the tattoo, a small cross on her outer ankle, when she visited some friends in a nearby city.

"Why didn't you ask me before you did it?" Mrs. Jones wanted to know.

"Mom, you would certainly have said 'no'. It's just cool, mom," was Diane's reply. "It doesn't mean that I belong to a gang or group. A small tattoo is the 'in thing' on college campuses. And it's nothing to be ashamed of, at all."

"Don't you know needles can transmit certain infections?" Mrs. Jones asked.

"I know. Mom, I did some homework. They used new needles every time and threw away the used ones. The tattoo apparatus was sterilized. I felt pretty safe."

"Well, why have God's symbol on your ankle?" Mrs. Jones asked next.

"Why not, Mom? You say God is everywhere. A cross in a chain around the neck, a cross in a bracelet; how are they different from the cross on my ankle?"

Mrs. Jones realized that she would not win this kind of argument. She said, "You're grownup now. You're smart. I feel you should not do anything to your body that causes permanent change. It's hard to remove a tattoo if you don't want it later."

Mrs. Jones came to my office and expressed concern about Diane. I consulted an infectious disease specialist, who said that it's not uncommon for young college students to get tattoos. Usually there are no problems, though problems do arise in other groups in our society, such as prisoners, who may have extensive tattoos. Members of those groups can have hepatitis B or C, AIDS, and other infections, the result of using drugs and indulging in indiscriminate sex. So far, there is no proof that tattooing alone causes AIDS or hepatitis when clean needles are used.

Diane had had hepatitis B shots before entering college. The specialist told me that if the parents were still worried, they could check Diane's blood for AIDS and for hepatitis C. I conveyed this message to Mrs. Jones. Diane was smart; she had checked the tattoo parlor, and knew exactly what she was getting into. Not all teenagers do that. There is no state facility that monitors the cleanliness of tattoo parlors or checks the qualifications of their employees. If needles are unclean, one can get serious life-threatening infections. Once the glamour of the tattoos fades away, they are not easy to remove.

Teenagers enjoy a lot of freedom in this country; that is the way it should be. But they need to remember that while fire cooks, it can also burn if one is not careful. Freedom is like a flame. One must use it very wisely.

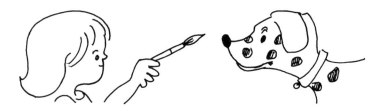

Body Piercing and Infections

aula, an 18-year-old, came to my office with a sore throat; she was also running a mild fever. While examining her I noticed that she had a navel ring and the area around the pierced navel site was red. The rest of her examination was normal.

"When did you get the navel ring?" I asked.

"A couple of weeks ago," she replied.

"Paula, it looks like it's getting infected," I told her. "I'm more worried about this than I am about the sore throat."

Paula's mother was upset because she didn't know that Paula had pierced her navel. "See how things can go wrong?" she commented as she looked at Paula.

Body piercing has become common among teenagers either for rebellious or cosmetic reasons. We don't have statistics pertaining to the frequency and complications of body piercing, but for teenagers the rim of the ear and the navel are the most popular sites, followed by the eyebrow, tongue, lips, and nipple.

Usually, tattoo artists and employees in jewelry stores do body piercing; many of them are untrained and unqualified. Except in Oregon and Texas, there are no regulations to monitor the cleanliness of the piercing establishment, and there are no provisions for checking the qualifications of the people who body-pierce. Because it looks easy, sometimes friends do piercing on each other.

What are the complications? Bacterial infections are common. Ear rim piercing may lead to infections with a germ called pseudomonas, which is hard to treat; ear lobe piercing may cause streptococcus or staphylococcus infections. If the infection is not treated promptly, permanent disfigurement can result. However, after piercing, infection in the navel area is usually fungal and is very difficult to get rid of. When teenagers get body-pierced by friends, they are setting themselves up for more infections, because friends often do not sterilize instruments.

An allergic reaction to jewelry is also common, because most jewelry used in piercing is inappropriate. Jewelry made of gold or stainless steel causes the least problems.

Paula's infection seemed likely to be bacterial; I therefore gave her an antibiotic that was good for the sore throat as well, and assured her mother that the infection would go away.

"I've warned Paula about the dangers of body piercing," I told her. "She is an adult now and understands the implications of her actions. This piercing bit is probably a passing fad; if she doesn't like the navel ring, she can easily get it removed later. Take it easy, though; raising children nowadays is like driving through heavy traffic. If you want to stay sane and avoid problems, sometimes it's best to go with the flow."

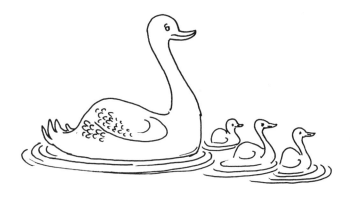

Bullying in Schools

*A*nita, a fifth grade student, came to my office with recurrent headaches and stomach pains. These complaints were noticed mostly on weekdays. Routine laboratory tests did not reveal any obvious cause, and after much goading, Anita confided that one of her classmates, Susie, bothered her at school. Susie was a bully who grabbed Anita's books and pencils without asking, bumped into her wantonly, and pushed her when the teacher was not around. Moreover, Susie had warned Anita that she "would get her" if she told on her to the teacher. Anita was upset about the whole situation and was scared to go to school.

Bullying, which is very common in schools, involves physical and/or psychological harassment of one student by another, through such means as hitting, pushing, belittling, and even the spreading of rumors. Twenty percent of students in grades six to ten are involved in bullying either as a bully or as a victim. In a study published in JAMA, the Journal of the American Medical Association, 15,000 students from private and public schools were interviewed. Out of them, 13 percent were bullies, 6.3 percent were victims, and 6.3 were both bullies and victims.

Bullying involves a bully, a victim, and bystanders. Bullies crave recognition, status, and power, so they need an audience as well as a victim. Without an audience there is no bully. For their part, bystanders generally have mixed feelings. They identify with the bully, indirectly enacting their own hidden yearning for power and recognition through the bully. They also identify with the victim and the consequent hurt; hence they don't join in bullying the victim. And because they are afraid, they don't report the bully to the school authorities.

In the JAMA study, bullies and their victims showed poor psychosocial functioning when compared to normal students. The bullies had negative attitudes towards school, poorer academics, and difficulty in making friends. Later in life, they were more prone to alcohol and tobacco abuse. Victims also had difficulty making friends. Students who were both bullies and victims often were depressed. An analysis of recent school shooting incidents has revealed issues of bullying and revenge.

What can be done about the prevalent school problem? A few schools in the United States have started a proactive team approach called a "Bully Task Force". Meeting regularly with a group of known bullies, their victims, and bystanders, it conducts classes about the mechanics of bullying, its effect on the victims, and the psychological factors involved. Students are encouraged to vent their feelings, and to discuss openly their roles in the bully-victim-bystander scenario. The bullies are encouraged to imagine themselves as victims and express their feelings in that role. When bullies empathize, their bullying behavior diminishes. The task force also suggests alternate ways they can handle frustration and feelings of inadequacy.

Every school should have a committee like the bully task force with teachers, parents, and a psychologist as members to handle bully problems and maintain a school environment that is physically and emotionally safe.

I advised Anita's mother to talk to the teacher and the school principal. Anita was transferred to another class section and did well.

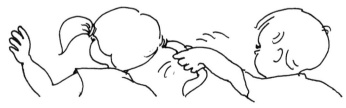

The Internet, Both Boon and Bane

Ed, 15 years old, loves the Internet, spending three or more hours a day in front of a computer. If asked, he tells his mother that he is working on a school project, but his grades are falling; moreover, he is putting on weight. Ed's mother is worried and expressed her concerns to me during one of the office visits.

Many parents feel comfortable and satisfied that their children are not watching much television but spending quality time in front of a computer. They will be surprised to know what some children do on the internet. No doubt there is much useful information available on the net but information that is detrimental is also there in plenty. Adolescents download violent games, sexy pictures and videos, and participate in chat groups, just to kill time. Shady characters solicit sex on the net. All these activities are detrimental to normal child development.

Long hours on the internet impede a child's development of social and interpersonal interactions with other family members, which may lead to poor social skills later on in life. Children fail to develop cooperation with others and do not understand healthy competition. They may suffer from emotional and social dysfunction and may turn unduly aggressive.

Video games in which players get involved in shooting and mutilation are used to train and desensitize troops for war. Children who participate in such games are rewarded with points for killing as many characters as possible, ostensibly without negative emotional consequences—but negative emotional consequences do occur.

The increase in violent crimes and school shootings is partly due to the availability of violent video games commercially and on the Internet. Young children and even a few adolescents do not understand the consequences of violence, and the emotional and financial toll it takes on the families.

Adolescents are constantly exposed to a barrage of junk e-mail. The University of New Hampshire "Crimes against Children" Research Center surveyed teens about unsolicited e-mail. Twenty-five percent of the teens reported that they had received e-mail with violent and sexual contents. Pictures of child pornography and letters soliciting sex are just a mouse-click away. These e-mails confuse children and teens and they lose their sense of security and reality.

The New Hampshire study also found that 20 percent of children were solicited for sex over the Internet. In 15 percent of those cases, the solicitor tried to contact the youngster either by phone or in person. The unsuspecting children had given out personal information such as age, address, and phone number to chat groups. The solicitor accessed the information, acted like a concerned adult or friend, and lured the youngster to a hotel or house on a false pretext. Such predators have killed a few children.

What should parents do? I told Ed's mother what I tell other parents: Your children know more than you think you know. They can conceal their activities on the Internet. So, to exercise parental control:

- Place the computer in a public area of the house where you can monitor your children's activities.
- Check often what they watch.
- Ask questions and make sure you look at the school assignments your children say they are doing on the Internet.
- Limit use of the Internet to about two hours a day.
- Tell your children not to provide any personal information on the net, and not to respond to unsolicited e-mail.

Baby's Baby

When I walked into the room, fifteen-year-old Tricia was trying to change her baby's diaper. Sara was crying and kicking her legs vigorously. As Tricia fastened one side of the tape of the diaper, the other end came off promptly. Tricia struggled to keep Sara's legs in position, and with a little help from me, finally succeeded in putting the diaper on.

"See, Doctor? She's a handful. I want to keep her dry, but she doesn't cooperate."

"How can you expect a four week old baby to cooperate?" I asked.

"I don't know. I brought her in today because she does not feed properly. She sucks for a minute and stops," said Tricia.

I examined Sara. She was healthy. "How often do you feed Sara and how much?" I asked.

"Every hour. She takes an ounce or two and stops. I don't know what's wrong with her." Tricia stuck the bottle in Sara's mouth, but the baby refused to suck. A little formula drooled out. "See? She's spitting."

"Do you have help at home?" I asked.

"I'm living with my mom. My mom and my boyfriend's mom give me advice," said Tricia. "My mom told me this milk formula doesn't suit Sara and wanted me to change to a soy formula. I tried soy milk for a day and the baby spat it up. Then my boyfriend's mother told me to give Nutramigen to Sara, but she spat that up, too. Now my mom is telling me to try goat's milk. I don't know what to do. I'm confused."

Tricia didn't know the proper technique of feeding and was

giving her baby too much formula. I told her to continue giving Nutramigen, two to four ounces every two and a half to three hours, and burp the baby after feeding. "When she cries don't give her the bottle every time; maybe she needs to be carried and hugged. Raising a child involves time and patience," I advised her.

Tricia was caught between her mother and her boyfriend's mother, both of whom gave her conflicting advice. Her boyfriend didn't get involved in making decisions except the one that produced Sara. He and Tricia either didn't know about or never considered contraception. They never seriously thought that their relationship would result in a child. When Sara was born, Tricia was ill-prepared and didn't even know how to change a diaper, or how to feed or cajole a baby. She wasn't emotionally mature enough to have a child. Emotionally, Tricia herself was a baby.

Approximately one million teenagers become pregnant each year in the United States. About 51 percent of teenage pregnancies end in live births, 35 percent result in induced abortion, and 14 percent end in miscarriage or stillbirth. Although the pregnancies among 15 to 19-year olds have declined, they have remained stable for adolescents younger than 15 years, a worrisome fact. More than 90 percent of teenage pregnancies are unintended.

Teenage pregnancy is a big problem for the families involved, and also, socially and economically, a problem for our society. Pregnant teenagers don't seek prenatal checkups. Consequently, teen pregnancies incur a greater number of complications such as bleeding, infections, and high blood pressure. The newborns often have low birth weight. There is also a higher incidence of deaths among babies born to teenagers. Adolescent mothers are less likely to marry or finish high school and are more likely to be unemployed. Children born to teenage mothers have more accidents at home and are more likely to be hospitalized before the age of five years.

What can we do to prevent teenage pregnancy? We need to provide both education and guidance. Approximately 25 percent of youth have had intercourse by 15 years of age. About 56 percent of girls and 73 percent of boys are sexually active before they reach 18. Doctors should encourage teenagers to postpone early sexual activity. Teenagers who are sexually active should be advised to try contraception. Parents should discuss with children, at appropriate ages, the emotional, economic, and social implications of teen pregnancy.

Approximately one-third of teenagers who become pregnant were themselves the product of a teenage pregnancy, so education includes setting a good example. Relatives and friends, school, church, doctors, and the media should communicate with teenagers and make them aware of the consequences of teenage pregnancy. It is, truly, everybody's responsibility.

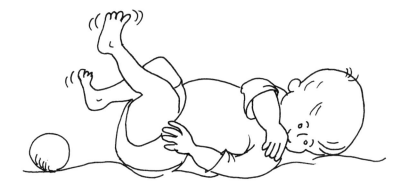

Be Careful Under the Mistletoe!

Chris, a teenager, had infectious mononucleosis. This disease causes weakness, fever, sore throat, and enlargement of the liver, spleen, and lymph glands.

"Chris, did you kiss anyone in the past few weeks?" I asked. Chris blushed. He had a girlfriend. He assured me that she did not have any signs or symptoms of mononucleosis.

A virus called Epstein-Barr virus (EBV) causes this disease. In children, transmission takes place through saliva by way of contaminated toys, pacifiers, bottles, and other objects. In young adults the virus is transmitted while kissing. EBV is excreted in the saliva before and during the disease period and sometimes up to six months after recovery.

There are many other diseases that are transmitted by saliva. Kissing can easily transmit bacterial diseases, such as streptococcal, pneumococcal, and meningococcal infections, as well as the common cold and flu.

Herpes Simplex (HSV 1), which causes fever blisters and mouth ulcers, is easily transmitted by kissing and through contaminated objects. The virus is found in the saliva of from 2 to 9 percent of adults and 5 to 8 percent of children.

The mumps virus also thrives in the saliva, which is infectious six days before the onset of the characteristic mumps' swelling. The virus has been detected in saliva up to two weeks after the swelling's onset.

The rabies virus has also been isolated in the saliva of people with rabies. However, there are no reported cases of people acquiring rabies just by kissing. Similarly, even though the AIDS virus is found in saliva, to date there have been no reports of the disease being transmitted by kissing.

A virus called Human Herpes Virus 8 (HHV-8) can cause a serious problem, especially to people with impaired immunity. This virus is found in the saliva of infected individuals and is transmitted to others by kissing; it causes a cancer called Kaposi's sarcoma and is also probably responsible for some tumors of the blood and lymph glands. In healthy individuals, the incidence of Kaposi's sarcoma is about 1 in 1000; however, in people with a poor immune system, such as those with AIDS or immune deficiencies, and in individuals on chemotherapy for cancers or with organ transplants, the HHV-8 causes Kaposi's sarcoma with an incidence as high as 50 percent. For such people, kissing could be very dangerous.

Am I scaring you? Kissing has health benefits too. Kissing is the key that unlocks love. It relieves stress by releasing mood-elevating chemicals called endorphins. It burns two calories per minute and firms your face muscles. That is something if you are a couch potato!

Chris recovered from his infection. Luckily, his girlfriend did not get infectious mononucleosis. All's well that ends well!

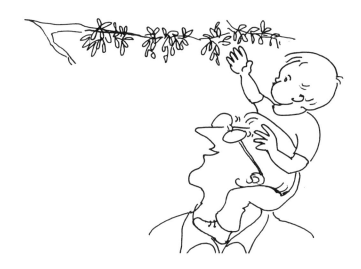

How Much of Your Life Do You Want to Lose?

I have known Joe since he was a child; I've seen him grow into a tall and handsome teenager of 17. One day Joe walked into my office complaining of an intermittent cough that became more intense at night. He was using Ventolin inhalers to get some relief.

During the physical examination, I could smell that he smoked. I heard wheezing in his chest. It was obvious that he had asthma that was made worse by his smoking.

"Joe," I told him, "I'll give you medications for your asthma. But they won't help you as long as you smoke."

"I know," he replied.

"Smoking aggravates asthma and leads to chronic lung disease," I went on. "In the long run it causes cancer of the lungs, esophagus, and stomach. It increases the risk of heart attacks and strokes."

"I know," said Joe.

"Then, why do you smoke?" I asked.

"Because it's cool! All my friends do it," Joe said. "I tried to stop, but I couldn't."

That is the problem. Peer pressure and the addictive nature of nicotine in cigarettes make it hard to give up smoking. Teenage smoking has risen alarmingly for the past four years. More than 20 percent of high school seniors smoke daily. Sixty percent of adult smokers became addicted by age 14, and 90 percent by age 18. It is the single most significant public health problem facing us today.

The statistics are appalling. Each year, smoking kills more

Americans than automobile accidents, AIDS, alcohol, cocaine, heroin, fires, homicides, and suicides, all combined. An estimated 3,000 teenagers start smoking each day, and about one-third eventually will die from a smoking-related illness. This translates into three million teenage smokers currently in this country, out of whom one million will die due to illnesses caused by smoking.

With all this information available, why do teenagers smoke? Peer pressure, poor self-image and the addictive nature of nicotine are the main causes. Parents who smoke, family problems, and sleek cigarette advertisements encourage teenage smoking. Movie stars and superstar players who smoke are not setting good examples. For many children, they are the role models. At one pack of cigarettes a day, an estimated four years of life is cut short. At two packs a day, eight years of one's life is lost. Long-term exposure to cigarette smoke from others causes 3,000 deaths a year in people who did not even touch a cigarette.

"Joe," I said, "you understand the terrible consequences of smoking. Your asthma won't get better if you don't stop smoking. Moreover, teenage boys who continue smoking through adulthood are about 50 percent more likely to become impotent than non-smokers. I want you to think about this."

That got Joe's attention. "I'll try harder to stop smoking," he said. As he left the room I gave him a copy of a rap song I wrote for elementary school students.

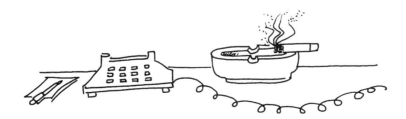

Listen to me, Don't be a fool!

Listen to me—don't be a fool,
Cigarette smoking is not cool!

Smoking causes high blood pressure;
Say 'no, no' to a friend's peer pressure.
Heart attacks are more when you smoke;
Don't let life go up in smoke!

Listen to me. Don't be a fool,
Cigarette smoking is not cool!

Mark my words, I'm telling you the truth,
Smoking causes stains on the tooth.
Cancer of the mouth, cancer of the throat,
Cancer of the lungs – are nothing to gloat!

Listen to me. Don't be a fool!
Cigarette smoking is not cool!

Smoking cuts your competence.
Boys may end with impotence.
Nicotine causes addiction
With hundred percent prediction!

Listen to me—Don't be a fool,
Cigarette smoking is not cool!

Smoking causes lung diseases.
Sooner than normal, all life ceases;
One pack a day will cut your life
By four full years—just like a knife!

Listen to me—Don't be a fool!
Cigarette smoking is not cool!

In smoke, untold chemicals are there;
All are poisons—be aware!
Children suffer when families smoke
Asthma, earaches—that's not a joke!

Listen to me—Don't be a foo!!
Cigarette smoking is not cool!

When friends smoke, you inhale
You have problems on a large scale.
Smoke is a poison; who needs it?
Tell your friends—ask them to quit!

Listen to me—Don't be a fool,
Cigarette smoking is not cool!

Asthma, wheezing, cough, and phlegm
Sooner or later you get them.
Smoking leads you straight to the grave.
Say no to smoking and be brave!

Listen to me—Don't be a fool!
Cigarette smoking is not cool!

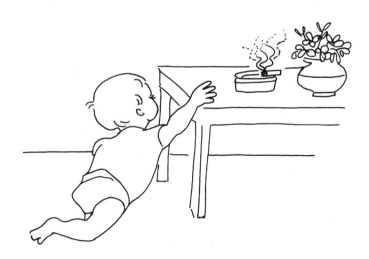

Rules Learned in Kindergarten

Four-year-old David was brought to my office by his mother after he had been exposed at a daycare center to a child having hepatitis. The daycare personnel were not sure what type of hepatitis the other child had.

David's physical examination was normal. As hepatitis A is more frequently seen at his age than other types of hepatic infections, I gave David an injection of human immune globulin as a preventive measure against that type. I informed his mother that the immune globulin was beneficial when given within 14 days of exposure to hepatitis A, and yet might not prevent the onset of the disease. We hoped for the best.

I saw David five days later. His appetite was gone and he felt weak. He had jaundice, a palpable liver with pain in that area, and his liver enzymes were high. A test for hepatitis A proved positive. Obviously, the immune globulin was given too late and David had developed full-blown hepatitis A.

Hepatitis A is a viral infection and the incubation period is 4 to 6 weeks. An infected child may not have any symptoms at all other than a mild cold. On the other hand, the child may have fever, weakness, nausea, vomiting, loss of appetite, abdominal pain, or jaundice. Adolescents may get depressed and may have general discontent, which has led to the cliché, "a jaundiced view of life." After several days or weeks, the child generally recovers. David recovered completely within only a couple of weeks, without complications.

How is hepatitis A transmitted? Even though contaminated foods and water have caused epidemics, this is not the usual way the disease spreads. In this country, daycare centers and households have become an important source for the spread of hepatitis A. The disease spreads through fecal contamination of bottles, spoons, toys, and other common objects that the child comes into oral contact with. It is a "fecal-oral route" disease. Sometimes, daycare personnel have a mild fever or cold and spread the disease to children in their care without realizing that they themselves have hepatitis A.

How can we prevent the spread of hepatitis A? By educating employees and family members about fecal-oral transmission. It is important to wash one's hands vigorously after changing diapers, and also before preparing and serving food. Because the hepatitis virus can survive for weeks on objects such as diaper-changing surfaces, toilet training equipment, toys, and sleeping equipment, these too must be kept meticulously clean.

Children and adults exposed to hepatitis A should receive immune globulin as soon as possible to prevent the onset of the disease. Now, a vaccine is available.

Many years ago my daughters' kindergarten teacher taught them a few rules. They were: clean up your mess, flush the toilet, wash your hands thoroughly before you eat, and so on. Just the rules needed to prevent the spread of hepatitis A!

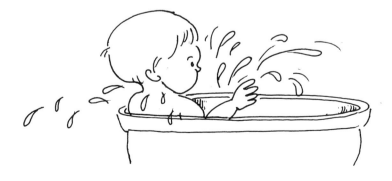

A Preventable Accident

I have known Eric since he was born. It was always a pleasure to check him as he was naturally cheerful and playful; however, his playfulness got him into trouble when he was four years old.

Eric had been playing with a nail and poked his left eye accidentally. Tears flowed profusely and he had intense pain; he could not see with his left eye and was rushed to the emergency room. We used fluorescein, a dye that sticks to the injured tissue, especially in the eye. When viewed under ultraviolet light, damage to the eye can be clearly seen, especially in the area over the cornea. Eric had a laceration of about 1 cm starting from the center of the cornea to the white portion of the eye called the sclera. Part of the lens material was torn off and oozed through the wound along with fluids of the eye. A CAT scan of the eye showed possible bleeding in the eye chambers and damage to the front portion of the eye.

This was bad news. An ophthalmologist was consulted.

Eric was started on intravenous antibiotics and taken to surgery. Already some pus had accumulated in the front chamber of the bloody eye. After putting some antibiotics into the eye, the specialist made delicate sutures in the cornea. We hoped for the best, but alas, the injury was extensive; the wound healed with shrinking and extensive scarring of the eye, ending in a total loss of vision in the left eye. Later when I saw Eric in my office I felt sorry for him, but he was as cheerful as ever.

Eye injury is a major cause of unilateral blindness in children. Annually there are about 2.4 million eye injuries in this country, and of this number up to 70,000 children develop some loss of vision. This statistic is appalling; it is sad when we realize that 90 percent of these eye injuries are preventable.

How do you prevent ocular injuries? At home, keep sharp objects, matches, and also chemicals such as detergents, spray cans, and ammonia away from children. When a chemical like a detergent falls in the eye, immediately wash the eye with warm tap water for at least twenty minutes. Make sure the water washes the inside of the eye, not just the lids. Simultaneously, contact your doctor.

If a large particle in the eye moves every time the child blinks, it may come out with tears or by washing the eye. If the particle does not flush out, take your child to the doctor.

In selecting toys for your child, buy only those that are age-appropriate. Avoid toys with sharp edges and pointed ends. Older children at home may be using darts and BB guns, so they should be educated in their safe use. BB gun pellets are notorious in causing blindness, so keep these guns away from younger children.

If you must set off fireworks near children, make sure that they and you all wear protective goggles.

Power lawn mowers eject small pebbles at high speeds and can cause severe damage to the eyes. Be careful while mowing the lawn, especially when children are around. Teach your children to wear protective goggles in laboratories, auto-welding workshops, etc.

Remember that 50 percent of eye injuries happen around the home and 90 percent of these injuries are preventable. Whenever I see Eric I always think that his blindness in one eye need not have happened at all.

 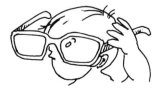

When Sweet Vitamins Can Harm

*T*hree-year-old Pamela often came to my office. She was cute and smart. As many children do, she hated to take medications. Her mother gave Pamela a chewable vitamin tablet every day, telling her it was candy; otherwise, Pamela refused to take it.

One day, Pamela was probably hungry and decided to have some candy. She moved a chair near the cabinet, climbed up, and grabbed the vitamin bottle. The childproof cap was not a problem, as Pamela had seen her mother open it many times. One by one she ate the vitamin tablets. After a while she vomited, attracting her mother's attention. The vomit smelled of vitamins; moreover, Pamela's mother noticed the empty vitamin bottle on the floor; that was when she called me.

Pamela had eaten about 40 vitamin tablets. These tablets had 12 mgs of iron fumarate in each one of them and Pamela had ingested a total of about 480 mgs of the iron salt in a single dose. That was iron poisoning! Pamela was rushed to the emergency room, where a tube was inserted into her stomach and the remaining vitamins and iron were washed out. A medication called deferoxamine, which binds iron to make it nontoxic, was put into her stomach. Because the serum iron level was high, I admitted Pamela to the hospital and she was given some more deferoxamine to flush out the excess iron from her blood.

Iron poisoning irritates the stomach and intestines causing abdominal pain, vomiting, diarrhea, and sometimes bleeding. Excessive amounts of iron cause cellular damage, especially in the liver, producing multiple late effects including death. I gave Pamela several blood tests to detect any delayed damage. I am glad to report that there was no permanent damage and Pamela recovered completely.

Childhood poisoning is common and preventable. Here are five simple steps you should take:

1. Keep medications in child safety bottles in cabinets beyond the reach of children, and install cabinet locks.
2. Keep only the medications that are needed and throw away the rest, including those that have expired.
3. Stick the number of the local poison control center on your phone.
4. Have a small bottle of syrup of ipecac handy in case your doctor advises you to induce vomiting.
5. Above all, don't tell children that a medicine is candy or grape juice, even though it tastes like it. Remember it is so easy to get poisoned by eating seemingly innocent tablets like multivitamins with iron.

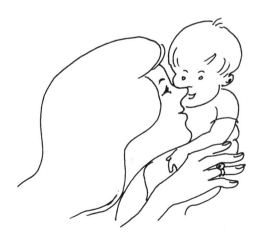

Life-Saving Advice

Five-year-old Shawn was rushed to the emergency room with his head and flank covered with clotted blood; he was unconscious and breathing hard. Immediately, the ER physician introduced a tube into his windpipe to administer oxygen. Simultaneously, a nurse started intravenous fluids. They rushed Shawn to the radiology department for a chest x-ray and a CAT scan of the head. The x-ray showed the presence of air between the chest wall and lungs, a condition called a pneumothorax. Air in that space would collapse the lungs and cause severe respiratory problems. The ER physician dexterously inserted a tube in Shawn's chest and drained the air. The CAT scan of the head showed a long skull fracture with bleeding in the covering layers of Shawn's brain and his cerebellum. The brain was swollen, a condition called cerebral edema. After stabilizing him, the ER physician transferred Shawn to a children's hospital.

Shawn was admitted to the pediatric intensive care unit. His pupils were different sizes, which indicated an increase in intracranial pressure. A neurosurgeon was consulted. Because Shawn's brain swelling did not become worse, the neurosurgeon advised a conservative treatment; Shawn was still unconscious, so a machine breathed for him, and intravenous fluids gave him nourishment.

In two days Shawn slowly came out of the coma. First, he could not speak, but with physiotherapy and continued medical management, he improved slowly. In six days, he was able to get up and take a few steps. He could eat pureed food and swallow fluids without choking.

Twenty days later, Shawn was discharged from the hospital.

At the time of discharge, he still had impaired cognition. He required supervision while walking and doing other activities.

Shawn is about ten years old now. He does not sleep well, has speech problems, and attends a special education class. He has behavioral problems of aggression and is being counseled. All these effects are due to the severe injuries that Shawn received to his brain earlier in his life.

How did Shawn sustain such a severe brain injury? Shawn and his sister were sitting in the front seat of a pickup truck driven by his father, and they were not wearing seat belts. When the truck rolled over, Shawn was ejected at 55 miles per hour and crashed unconscious on to the road.

Please buckle up all your loved ones when you drive, and be sure to buckle up yourself.

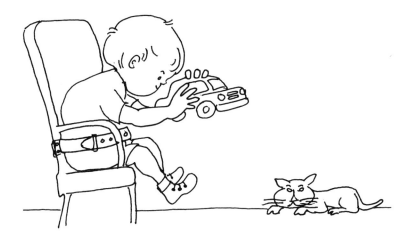

Preventing Shaken Baby Syndrome

I first saw Miguel Guerrero when he was a month and half old. He had profuse hair, black as India ink, and almond eyes. On examination I found a minimal collection of fluid in his scrotum, a condition called "hydrocele" that spontaneously resolved itself in a few weeks. Later I took care of his sore throats and ear infections, and gave him routine immunizations. At the age of two years he weighed a chubby twenty-eight pounds. Active and full of smiles, he was a joy to his parents.

Early one morning, the Guerreros dropped Miguel and his four-year-old brother off at the baby sitter on their way to work, with lots of bye-byes and kisses. When they came back, they learned that Miguel had been injured and was in the emergency room of a local hospital. The baby sitter said he had dropped Miguel accidentally; when the child did not breathe, the sitter's wife gave him CPR and called an ambulance.

Miguel was unconscious, had a stiff neck, and curved his body backward; all this indicated a severe brain injury. As he was not breathing, he was intubated and oxygen was given by a respirator. Then he was transferred to a children's hospital.

A CAT scan on Miguel revealed minimal bleeding in the meninges, the covering membrane of his brain. The brain has cavities known as ventricles that are filled with a liquid, the cerebrospinal fluid (CSF). Imagine a tender coconut: The outer hard shell is the skull, the brown layer covering the kernel is the meninges; the white kernel is the brain; and the cavity and the coconut water represent the ventricle and CSF.

Due to the injury, the CSF was not circulating properly in

Miguel's brain. In addition, the brain tissue swelled up, resulting in increased pressure inside the brain. To reduce the pressure, a neurosurgeon introduced one end of a thin tube into Miguel's ventricle and placed the other end inside his abdominal cavity. This device, a ventriculo-peritoneal shunt, drains the CSF from the brain into the abdominal cavity. It promptly reduced Miguel's intracranial pressure.

Miguel had several other complications. He aspirated mucous or food while unconscious and developed pneumonia in his lungs. He had bleeding in retina. He developed meningitis and severe seizures, which were controlled by medications.

Children fall or accidentally get dropped; usually they don't get hurt seriously. The presence of bleeding in the brain and retina, however, suggest a serious injury such as happens when a child is violently shaken. When shaken thus, the brain bounces back and forth inside the skull and hits against the skull bones, which results in bleeding and brain damage. This form injury is called the "shaken baby syndrome."

Shaken baby syndrome is a form of child abuse. It is seen in children younger than three years of age; most cases happen during the first year of life. The child may exhibit lethargy, impaired consciousness, poor feeding, breathing difficulty, or neurologic manifestations. The child may develop seizures, lapse into a coma, and die. According to Dr. Ann-Christine Duhaime of Children's Hospital of Philadelphia, child abuse involving head injuries causes more deaths than injuries to other body parts.

Parents may shake their children or toss them up and down unaware of the hidden danger.

Parents or a baby sitter may shake a crying child to calm him or her down. Occasionally an adult gets angry, impatient, or frustrated, and takes it out on the child. More often, this happens with young parents or baby sitters, unstable family situations, low socioeconomic conditions and with a premature or handicapped child. The perpetrators often deny that they had shaken the child.

So what should you do? Don't toss your child up and down or shake the child even playfully. If you leave your child with baby sitters, make them aware of this syndrome. Talk to other mothers about any misgivings they may have with baby sitters or day care personnel. If you notice any suspicious bumps or bruises, do not ignore them but take your child to a doctor. If uncomfortable with your baby sitter, look for another one.

Miguel is developmentally disabled, can't walk or talk, and is visually handicapped. He has a small feeding hole over his abdomen for pumping formula in. He is beginning to swallow pureed foods slowly. Even though Miguel won't be back to normal because of the brain injury, his mother believes he will recover completely one day. That is how mothers are, always hoping for the best for their children.

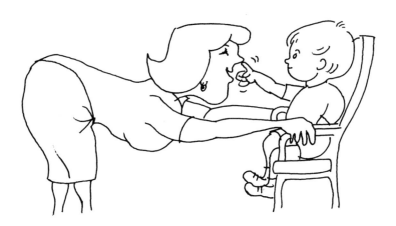

A Year Too Late

*J*ose's mother carried her son into my office and wanted him to be seen immediately. One look at her swollen red eyes told me that she had had a sleepless, worrisome night. I dropped what I was doing and rushed into the examining room. Jose was three years old and I had seen him several times, playful and always happy. But that day he was listless and limp. In between sobs, his mother told me the story.

The runny nose had started three days earlier. First she thought it was the usual common cold, but the next day he spiked a fever. She called her husband and told him that maybe she should take Jose to the doctor. Her husband, a salesman always on the move, decided that it was nothing serious because it was the "flu" season and he advised her to give the child Tylenol. Jose stopped eating and taking fluids. Bright light hurt his eyes. He lost interest in his favorite GI Joe toy and later even forgot the toy's name. He complained of a severe headache, vomited a couple of times, and lay still. His mother realized something was terribly wrong and brought him to my office.

As I examined him, Jose didn't recognize me. He had an ear infection and a sore throat. I tried to bend his neck, but it was like hardboard. Normally, I would be able to bend his neck so that the chin touches the chest. In other words, Jose had nuchal rigidity. This was a serious finding, which indicated that Jose had meningitis, an infection of the covering of the brain.

There was no time to lose. We rushed him to the emergency room, and a lumbar puncture was performed. This is a technique of just taking a few milliliters of cerebrospinal fluid from the covering space of the spinal cord for analysis. The fluid was turbid, indicating an infection. Immediately, a large dose of an antibiotic was given intravenously. Within a few minutes, I received the results of the test. The fluid was full of pus cells. Staining the fluid revealed the presence of variously shaped organisms.

Several years ago, we had to wait for a couple of days to identify the germs causing such an infection. Now, we have sophisticated techniques that can identify these germs within a few minutes. A test called "latex agglutination" showed that Jose had an infection due to a germ called "H. influenzae", belonging to the type b subgroup.

This is a serious infection. It may start out as a cold or cough and may lead to an ear infection, pneumonia or meningitis. Some people carry this germ. Children in nursery schools and daycare centers are particularly vulnerable. In this country, H. influenzae type b meningitis used to be the leading cause of death in children between the ages of one month and four years, and the incidence was 3 to 7 children per 100,000. If treated early, many children recover from meningitis. But the disease still takes its toll: some children still develop deafness, learning disabilities, weakness, seizures, and even mental retardation after recovering from meningitis.

Jose developed seizures. We gave intravenous anticonvulsants, adjusted his electrolytes, and maintained his oxygenation. As this was getting too complicated, I transferred him to the Intensive Care Unit of a nearby children's hospital. In a few hours, alas, Jose went into a deep coma and died.

I went ahead and prescribed antibiotics to the siblings. The parents of the children who came into contact with Jose were urged to see their own pediatricians for appropriate treatment.

Sorrow at the loss of Jose, and possibly feelings of guilt that she did not bring him earlier to be checked, made his mother's life miserable for a few months. Moreover, she and her husband blamed each other for the demise of Jose. I suggested psychological counseling, and consoled her, explaining that it had been a bad infection that, in spite of our best efforts, had ended adversely. However, she continued to mourn.

Time is the best healer of wounds of the body and the soul; she had another son, saw Jose in him, and got over her grief.

Is this infection curable? Yes, it is, if it is diagnosed early. Better than that, this infection is preventable, because we now have various vaccines available against this disease. Ninety-nine percent of the children thus vaccinated are protected. This is quite a breakthrough in the history of the prevention of diseases.

Hence I urge all parents to take their children in to the doctor's office for proper vaccination against this dreadful disease. But, alas, as fate would have it, this vaccine was introduced about a year after Jose died.

One year too late!

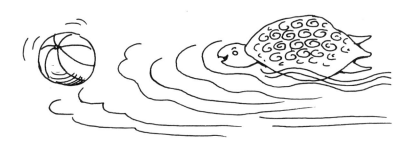

When a Child Bites

Bites are very common in children; in fact, they are the leading cause of injury in child-care centers in the United States. Early in life, biting is natural; young children keep all kinds of things in their mouth and bite on them as they explore their world. Some preschool and early grade schoolchildren resort to biting when they are unable to control their anger or cannot cope with a problem. Others, especially the youngest ones in a family, bite in order to gain power and thus control of a situation. Stress also leads to biting.

Some individuals even bite and self-mutilate themselves, as happens with those affected by a disease called Lesch-Nyhan syndrome. In a different context, patients who are upset may bite medical personnel. People bite each other while they fight. A bite injury can happen in yet another way, when a child or older person hits an opponent on the mouth with a clenched fist; and the teeth penetrate the hand, causing a wound. Here I must point out that not all bites are punitive, or result from aggression; some adult bites are just "love nips" bestowed by over-enthusiastic lovers on their partner's neck or private parts.

Whatever the cause, human bites are notoriously dangerous, more so than animal bites. This is because an individual's mouth is a cultural haven for bacteria such as streptococci, staphylococci, E. corrodens, and *fusobacterium nucleatum*, to name a few. Some bacteria need oxygen for their survival and are termed aerobic; others don't need oxygen, and are known as the anaerobic bacteria. You will be surprised to know that there are nooks and corners in our mouths where oxygen does not seep in; that is where the anaerobic bacteria thrive; they contaminate the bite wound and cause havoc if not treated promptly.

All human bites invariably get infected and need to be treated with antibiotics. Though tetanus rarely occurs after a human bite, the attacker may carry infections such as hepatitis B and C, or even HIV, and may occasionally transmit the disease through the bite. Your doctor may need to talk to the biter's parents or to their family doctor to run appropriate tests to detect such diseases. At the same time, the child or person who has been bitten also needs to be tested to make sure he or she does not already have the disease, which would put the biter at risk.

If your child is a biter, you can help curb the behavior by firmly telling your child, "No, don't bite, it hurts." Provide a toddler with a teething toy or other things that he or she can bite to his or her heart's content. If the child is the youngest, make sure the older siblings are not picking on him or her. After a biting incident, remove the biter from the company of others, and stay with the child till he or she calms down. If a stressful situation precipitates the biting behavior, try to anticipate it and avoid putting your child in that predicament in future. Help your child to find other ways to express his or her feelings when coping with an unpleasant situation.

If a child is bitten and the bite site is bleeding, apply pressure to the site with a clean piece of cloth or bandage. If gloves are available, wear them to protect yourself against exposure to blood. Once the bleeding stops, clean the wound with soap and water. Dry the wound, cover it with a clean cloth and call your doctor. Keep your child's immunization record handy; your doctor may need it to update tetanus and hepatitis B immunizations. If the bleeding does not stop in ten minutes, you may want to take the child directly to the emergency room.

As a concerned parent, check your child's daycare center for adequate staffing; make sure staff members are reliable, vigilant, and aware of childhood injuries. Don't ignore any human bite however small it is, because they are all dangerous.

Biting episodes are common in institutions for developmentally disabled persons as well. Because of their handicap, these individuals easily get frustrated, sometimes engaging in these undesirable acts. Here, it is usually easy to get blood tests on the biter and the bitten for the diseases mentioned earlier.

Once I had a very interesting experience involving a bite in an institution for the elderly. I was asked to examine Mary, who had a bruise on her shoulder. Someone had bitten Mary and I could clearly see the tooth impressions above the bruise. The caretaker did not witness the incident, but suspected John, who was developmentally disabled and lived at the same institution. Did John do it?

I asked for several blood tests on Mary and John; they were negative for contagious diseases. Meanwhile, I asked a dentist whether he could take a dental mold on John, so that he could compare the teeth marks on Mary's shoulder with John's dental mold. After obtaining permission from John's conservator, the smart dentist did exactly what I had requested. The teeth marks on Mary matched John's dental mold; Columbo would have loved it!

Perhaps, with proper legal guidance, institutions such as nursing homes will be able to keep dental molds of potential biters on file. When a bite mark is noticed, a quick comparison of the bite mark with a dental mold will promptly point to the perpetrator; this in turn may prevent unnecessary investigations, and also, on occasion, disprove false allegations.

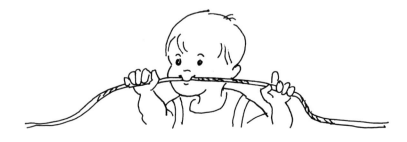

A Thanksgiving to Remember

"Dr. Rao, is it OK to eat turkey meat when a little bit of mercury was spilled on it?" Mrs. Baldwin casually asked me on the phone. I was working in the emergency room of a children's hospital.

"No, it's not safe to eat the turkey," I answered.

"It's too late in the evening to get another. How will I feed my friends and guests? Can't I scrape it off a little, clean it, and use it?" Mrs. Baldwin now seemed agitated.

"I'm sorry, Mrs. Baldwin. Tell me exactly what happened," I said.

"I placed the turkey in the oven. After a while, when I checked it, I thought it wasn't cooked thoroughly, so I shoved a mercury thermometer in, and the thermometer broke, spilling the mercury inside," she said. "I should have been more careful."

Celsius mercury thermometers were at one time frequently used to check temperatures in food, and if one broke, it posed a serious danger. True, liquid mercury is poorly absorbed when ingested, but mercury vaporizes readily when heated and it is then easily absorbed and can cause various problems such as weakness, chills, a metallic taste, nausea, vomiting, diarrhea, breathlessness, coughing, and a feeling of tightness in the chest. Pneumonitis and kidney problems have also been reported after a short exposure.

Children less than 30 months of age are very susceptible to mercury vapor toxicity. They can easily develop respiratory problems, eye irritation, and an itchy rash.

I told Mrs. Baldwin to open all the windows and turn on the exhaust fan immediately. I explained all the symptoms and signs of mercury vapor poisoning and requested her to bring her children to the emergency room if any symptoms developed. In addition to the mercury problem, there could be glass pieces in the turkey. I also told her she should discard the turkey at once in the garbage can, and place it outside the house.

"I feel bad that you don't have a turkey for Thanksgiving," I said, "but you know, it's better to be safe than sorry later."

"Doctor, that's OK," she said. "My children are fine. That itself is a Happy Thanksgiving for me!"

Though this incident happened many years ago, every Thanksgiving I invariably remember it.

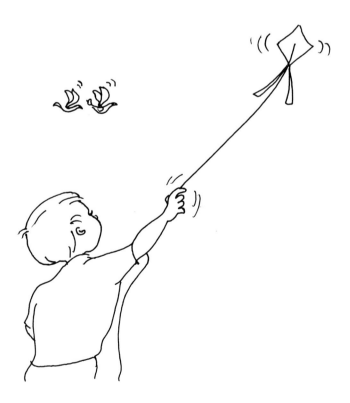

Superbugs and Superantibiotics

"Doc, Stephanie has a sore throat," said Mrs. Jeans. "I think she needs an antibiotic. Can you please prescribe one of the new ones she can take just once a day?"

Stephanie was five years old. She did not have a fever and was active and alert. Her throat was red, without pus pockets; the rest of her examination was normal.

"Stephanie has a sore throat, most likely due to a virus," I said.

"How do you know that?"

"Mrs. Jeans, a child with a bacterial infection usually has a high fever, headache, vomiting, and abdominal pain. Stephanie doesn't have these symptoms. More than seventy percent of sore throats with runny noses in children are due to viruses. I will give her a decongestant; she doesn't need an antibiotic. Believe me, by giving antibiotics indiscriminately, I will do more harm in the long run."

"Why is that, Doc?"

"Long-acting antibiotics, like the one you requested, are called broad spectrum antibiotics. They are very powerful and kill many varieties of germs. You can call them 'big guns'. The problem is that they destroy not just bad germs, but also the normal bacterial colonies that protect us against bad germs. Moreover, some germs have become immune to commonly used antibiotics like amoxicillin and also to some of the big gun antibiotics. These germs, one can call them superbugs, can spread and cause life-threatening infections."

"Superbugs!" she exclaimed, quite surprised. "Can you name a few?"

"Some pneumococci, which cause ear infections, pneumonia, blood infections, and meningitis; staphylococci, which cause abscesses; enterococci, which cause diarrhea and urinary tract infections; and bacteria that cause tuberculosis—all these have become resistant to multiple antibiotics. They can spread fast in schools and daycare centers. Can you imagine the havoc these bugs can cause?"

"How do these bacteria develop antibiotic resistance?" Mrs. Jeans asked.

"Random mutation can produce a drug-resistant germ that multiplies into millions in hours, passing on those genes to offspring. Some germs even develop enzymes that destroy the antibiotics. And there are many other ways."

"Will making even more powerful antibiotics resolve this problem?"

"As newer and stronger antibiotics become available, doctors will use them more, and germs will develop resistance to them as well. Do you know who'll win this war at the end? The germs! However, you parents can help prevent the creation of superbugs."

"Tell me how?"

"In several ways. Don't pressure us to prescribe an antibiotic; please leave that decision to doctors. When one is prescribed, finish the antibiotic. Don't stop when the child feels better, and don't give leftover antibiotics to another child, as inadequate treatment leads to increased bacterial resistance."

"Thank you, doctor; I didn't realize that taking an antibiotic when it wasn't needed could really harm my child," Mrs. Jeans replied. "Now that you've told me, I'll be sure to share that with my friends."

You'll be doing your friends and their children a favor, too, if you share this knowledge with them as well.

Dogs That Jump Over the Fence

As usual, Holly was plodding home from school with a backpack full of books. Her route lay around the corner store, alongside a fenced-in yard with a barking dog, and across a field with a few plum trees. Each day, as she passed by the fence, she teased the dog who, being chained, would go crazy and bark at her furiously. She thought this was fun, but one day either the fence was loose or the dog broke its chain; it came charging out and grabbed her ankle. Holly screamed, struggled, and somehow managed to shake him off and bolt to her house. The dog meanwhile, satisfied with the outcome, retreated behind the fence.

Holly was taken to the emergency room and had a few stitches put in over her ankle. I saw her next day. Her tetanus shots were up-to-date. While I tended to Holly's wounds, her Mom told me how Holly had received the injury.

I asked, "Do you know the owner of the dog? Did you talk to him?"

"I don't know him that well. He lives down the street."

"Did the dog have shots for rabies?"

"Yes, he said so. He said that Holly must have meddled with the dog somehow; he said he's a nice dog; wouldn't hurt a fly."

"That may be so, but did you notify the Humane Society so they can check the shot records?"

"No, I didn't. I was told that if the dog has had all the shots, there's no chance of Holly getting rabies."

"That's true. But did you ask the dog's owner to show you the vaccination papers? How are you sure that he even had the dog vaccinated? Don't misunderstand me. How are you sure he is telling the truth? If things go wrong, it's your child who will suffer."

"Well, I didn't think that far."

"The Humane Society, you know, would check the vaccinations; if they are not up-to-date, the owner should tie up the dog. If the dog is all right for 7 to 10 days, there is no cause to worry. Otherwise, I will be giving Holly a few shots to prevent rabies."

Holly's mother was very much concerned now, and we notified the Humane Society. I cleaned and dressed the wound, prescribed antibiotics, and sent Holly home.

The next day, a person from the Humane Society went to check on the dog. The dog's owner was home, but not the dog—the man said that the dog had jumped over the fence during the night and run away.

"Did the dog have rabies shots?" asked the Humane Society employee.

"I think so, but I'm not sure."

"Why aren't you sure?"

"The dog was given to me by a friend, who left for Mexico a few days ago."

"Do you have the shot records?"

"No, my friend didn't give me those papers."

"Can you contact your friend in Mexico?"

"No, he was a laborer and did not leave an address."

Rabies is a terrible disease. After being bitten by a rabid animal, a child develops lassitude, fever, a headache, and other symptoms that may look just like a common cold. After a period of about two to ten days, the child's attempts to swallow liquids, including saliva, result in spasms of the throat. The child can't swallow. Eventually, even the very sight of water evokes spasms, and this is called hydrophobia. Fanning a current of air across the face causes violent spasms of the throat and neck muscles. This is called "aerophobia". The child can't eat and drink and gets terrified. Soon, seizures develop, paralysis and coma follow, and the child dies due to the complications of the coma.

I have seen people suffer and die with rabies. Once you have seen such suffering, it is etched in one's memory forever.

I gave Holly the human rabies immune globulin and five shots of antirabies vaccine. Fortunately, she did fine.

If a cat or a dog or any animal bites your child, do not ignore it. If it happens to be someone else's pet, make sure to notify the Humane Society and at the same time seek prompt medical care. Not all people take proper care of their pets, and when they perceive problems arising because of their pets, they don't want to get involved. That's when the dog will magically jump over the fence and disappear!

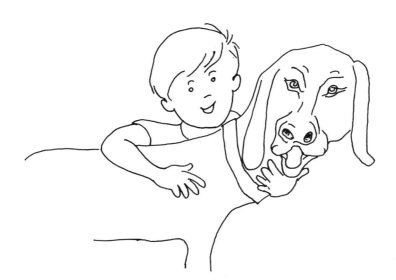

The "Longest Scar" Competition

*D*uke's teacher had announced a competition. "Who has the longest scar?" was the question. "You know, Dr. Rao, I got second place," said Duke with a broad smile, as I examined him one day. The scar he showed me was 6.75 inches long and 3/4 of an inch wide over his breastbone, or sternum.

"How did you get the scar?" I asked. Duke had a story to tell.

About four years ago, he and his brother were playing with a BB gun that could fire twelve shots, when the gun suddenly went off. Duke noticed blood oozing from his chest and panicked; he was rushed to the emergency room. X rays showed that a BB pellet had hit his sternum, ricocheted left, and become embedded in the pericardium, the sac surrounding his heart. Duke was extremely lucky because the pellet had stopped there and did not enter the heart. The situation was life threatening and he was taken to a nearby children's hospital.

Modern BB guns, otherwise called air guns, are very powerful. They can produce a muzzle velocity of 1,200 feet per second, which is faster than that produced by many low-velocity handguns. Hence BB guns have the ability to cause severe damage or death.

More than 30,000 BB gun injuries occur each year in this country. Boys aged 10 through 14 years run the highest risk of injury. Sixty-two percent of the injuries are unintentional, similar to Duke's incident; however, 13.7 percent are due to assault. In 1996, the surgery department of the University of Illinois at Chicago documented 16 patients who had severe assault BB gun injuries. Seven patients had injuries to the chest and back. In two patients the pellet had penetrated the aorta; one of the victims died. In another child the iliac artery and colon were damaged. Researchers analyzing the causes of the shootings were amazed because they happened after only minor arguments. The assailants were neighborhood children in seven cases, friends in five, and siblings in two incidents.

While BB pellets can injure various body parts, the eye is the organ most commonly injured, frequently resulting in blindness. Often the injured eye needs to be scooped out. Injuries to the head, carotid arteries, chest, heart, abdominal organs, and genitalia have all been described. In one incident the pellet had entered a blood vessel and caused an embolism.

What can we do about this problem? Parents should realize that BB guns are not toys. They should safely lock them up and allow children to use them only under strict supervision. Children should not be able to reach the guns impulsively, especially when they are angry or upset, because BB guns are increasingly being used for assault purposes or suicides. Schools and news media should warn children and adults about the dangers of guns.

Duke was operated on and the pellet was removed safely from his pericardium. The operation had left a long scar on his sternum, which won him a second place in the "longest scar competition."

While Duke was shot by his brother, ten-year-old David was injured by his neighbor's BB gun. A few days before he came to me, David had been running and playing in his neighborhood. That evening, his friend's father shot at a stray cat with his BB gun. Unfortunately, David ran between the cat and the gun and a pellet hit him in his face. He had intense pain and could not see, so his parents rushed him to a nearby emergency room. A CAT scan showed a ruptured eyeball with a pellet firmly lodged in the back of David's eye. The doctor gave him a shot of an antibiotic and pain medication, applied an eye patch, and transferred him to a children's hospital. There, an ophthalmologist performed a delicate operation and removed the BB pellet.

As I examined David several weeks later, I asked him, "Are you angry at the person who caused this injury?"

He answered without any hesitation, "No, doctor. It was just an accident."

I wish I had such a big heart. David is blind in his left eye.

Seeing the grave harm that this weapon can do, why do you need a BB gun at home?

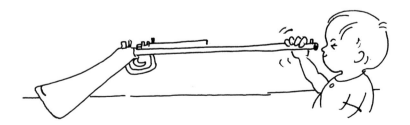

A Lesson from a Gopher

Cynthia was a lovely five-year-old girl. One day, when her father was mowing the lawn and chatting with her, a gopher fell in a small hole and was trying to get out. Cynthia's dad, a very kind man, did not want to kill the animal; instead, he went inside the house to get something with which to catch it, so he could free it in the fields later. Cynthia was left to watch the gopher that was trying hard to get out of the hole.

"You poor thing!" said Cynthia, and grabbed the creature to help it out. The 'poor thing' promptly bit her, jumped out, and disappeared in the grass. Cynthia's cries brought her father running out of the house; he drove her to my office for treatment.

Many television programs and children's books portray animals as lovable and harmless friends. Many parents assume that children are most likely to be bitten by strange or wild animals, but most bites are caused by family pets and other animals the child knows. So Cynthia's experience was unusual.

Several diseases can be transmitted to humans by animal bites. Bacterial infections, tetanus, and rabies are a few salient examples. Even a minor bite can lead to a serious infection, permanent damage, and emotional problems.

Rabies is a serious disease transmitted by the bite of animals. This disease affects the nervous system causing anxiety, difficulty in swallowing, paralysis, and seizures leading to death. Rabies is caused by a virus that lives in many wild animals such as bats, skunks, raccoons, and foxes. Small rodents, woodchucks, rabbits, and hares get infected by coming into contact with other wild animals. Sometimes the wild animals infect domestic dogs, cats, and ferrets.

The risk of contracting rabies depends on the animal. Bites from wild animals such as bats, raccoons, and skunks carry a high risk of rabies. Cats and dogs that have been immunized have a lower risk of rabies. For proper treatment of the child, doctors need to know whether the animal has rabies. The animal, if small, can be captured and confined for later examination by the health department or veterinarian. If the animal has been killed, its brain can be examined for rabies. A pet dog or cat can be tied up and observed for a period of ten days; if the animal remains healthy at the end of that time, there is no risk of rabies. Do not destroy the animal. I had a parent once who killed and buried a dog after it had bitten his child, thus destroying all evidence that it might have had rabies. As always, contact your doctor for advice.

Cynthia's tetanus immunization was current. I called the local health department personnel, and they advised me that rabies was never detected in gophers in the county where Cynthia lived. I prescribed an antibiotic to prevent serious infection; when I checked her after a week, she was doing well.

It is nice to be kind to animals, but children should be educated regarding appropriate behavior around family pets as well as strange animals.

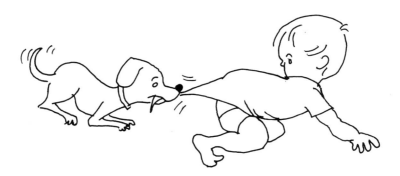

Children and Small Objects

I have known Angel Arias since his birth. Unfortunately, he had multiple problems during infancy. At six weeks of age, he had a lung infection and seizures, and his electrolytes were abnormal. All these medical problems affected him, so that at five years of age, he was behind in development when compared to other children his age.

One morning, when Angel had refused to eat and had vomited after eating solid foods, his mother brought him to my office. He was spitting out profuse amounts of mucous, and the more he spit, the more spit was formed. Angel was restless and very uncomfortable.

I learned from Mrs. Arias that Angel had a habit of eating small objects, a tendency called "pica". Angel was playing with toys that morning and it was possible that he could have swallowed a small piece of a toy, causing the problem.

Copious drooling with much discomfort in children usually indicates a foreign object stuck in the esophagus (food pipe). Usually these children will not be able to eat or drink; if swallowing solid foods or liquids is attempted, they will vomit. Angel could take a few sips of clear fluids, but not solid foods. That puzzled me.

X rays revealed a nickel lodged vertically in the upper part of Angel's esophagus. In that position, water could flow by the sides of the coin, but thicker foods could not pass; that's why Angel vomited only solid foods.

I consulted a gastroenterologist. The specialist removed the nickel with an endoscope under general anesthesia. The esophagus was not damaged, and Angel recovered completely.

It is common for children to ingest foreign materials. They swallow a variety of objects, such as coins, batteries, buttons, plastic toys, toy parts, safety pins, paint flakes, hair, and insects. Normally these objects pass into the stomach without causing any problems, but sometimes they can get stuck in the esophagus, which typically narrows in three places along its length.

Children are fascinated by round shining objects such as coins and small electrical batteries. Batteries are not waterproof, and saliva and other bodily secretions can enter them and liberate chemicals like potassium hypochloride, which can cause corrosive lesions. This may lead to a perforation of the esophagus, which could be fatal if it isn't recognized and treated promptly.

Children sustain many types of injuries, which vary according to the child's age. According to recent studies published in the Journal of Pediatrics, falls are the leading cause of injuries among children less than a year old. Falls from furniture are common between 6 to 8 months, and the swallowing of foreign materials between 9 to 11 months. The maximum number of childhood accidents occurs between 15 and 17 months of age.

Toddlers are also at risk for falls, drowning and burns. This is because at this age children acquire mobility and develop exploratory behavior. Kindergarten and elementary school children are more prone to bicycle, mini-scooter, and pedestrian injuries. Burns and drowning are also seen at this age group.

During teenage years, automobile injuries are more common. Self-inflicted injuries, burns, drowning, and firearm injuries are seen as well in this age group.

How do you prevent such injuries? Parents and others who care for children should assume responsibility to keep their children in infant car seats with restraints or seat belts while driving. They should provide bicycle helmets and insist that their children wear them. Other measures, such as installing a smoke detector at home, reducing the hot water temperature to avoid scalding, choosing proper furniture, using childproof caps to prevent accidental poisoning, and keeping firearms safe should all be encouraged.

To prevent foreign body ingestion and its complications, parents should give their children toys that are age-appropriate. They should make sure that the toys do not have small removable parts. With dolls, the buttons should not be loose. Some cuddly toys have attractive, plastic eyes, which children can pry open and swallow. Some toys have small batteries, and adults should make sure that children cannot get at them. Also, keep coins away from your little ones. As always, prevention is better than a cure!

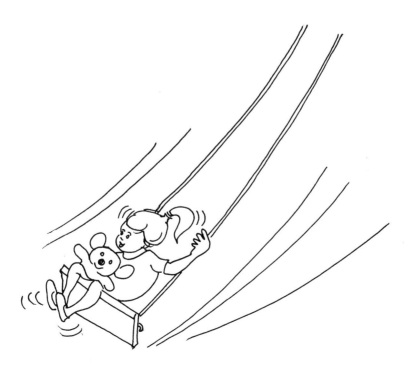

Monica's Malady

Mrs. Jacobs and her four-year-old daughter, Monica, lived in a small apartment. One day Mrs. Jacobs noticed a few cockroaches in her kitchen. She grabbed a can of roach killer and sprayed the entire house; then she forgot all about it.

After two months, Mrs. Jacobs noticed that Monica was looking pale and was bleeding from her gums. This worried her and she brought Monica to the hospital.

I found no family history of bleeding tendencies, or any similar illnesses. She was well nourished but looked pale. Her gums and cracked lips oozed small amounts of blood and her skin had small patches of blood accumulation called ecchymoses. Small lymph glands were noticed and the liver was just palpable. There were no bony abnormalities.

Lab tests revealed that Monica's hemoglobin, the pigment which carries oxygen from the lungs to all body parts, was a very low 4.5 grams percent, compared to about 11.5 to 15.5 grams percent normal for her age. Her white cells and platelets were also low. The decrease in platelets was the cause of her bleeding. Her bone marrow showed scanty red cell, white cell, and platelet precursors.

After eliminating many possibilities by appropriate tests, we arrived at a diagnosis of bone marrow aplasia; this meant that the marrow had totally shut down and was not producing any blood cells. If this condition persisted, Monica would succumb to complications of severe anemia, bleeding, or serious infection.

Bone marrow aplasia can be treated in several ways. After consulting experts, I started Monica on prednisone and an androgen preparation because these drugs stimulate bone marrow. After twelve weeks of treatment, her hemoglobin rose to 16.6 grams percent; her platelets and white cells also increased and reached normal levels, and she felt a lot better.

But a surprise awaited me. The hemoglobin which increased in Monica was not the usual adult hemoglobin (Hb A), but a variety called fetal hemoglobin (Hb F) that is normally present in fetuses and newborns, but decreases rapidly soon after birth. By the age of six to twelve months, almost 95 percent of the hemoglobin is of the adult variety. A few cells capable of producing Hb F still linger in the bone marrow and thus a small quantity of Hb F is found in adults. Luckily, the drugs I gave Monica had stimulated those latent Hb F producing cells. She didn't need a bone marrow transplant, but did need long-term therapy with hormones.

Bone marrow can shut down for any of several reasons. Drugs used in cancer treatment, antibiotics like chloramphenicol and sulfonamides, and seizure medications can cause this condition; radiation exposure, infections like viral hepatitis and infectious mononucleosis can also cause bone marrow to shut down. In about half the cases no cause is found, but chemical exposure is strongly suspected.

I feel that Monica probably got exposed to chemicals in the insecticide spray and developed severe anemia and bleeding problems. While using insecticides, parents should be aware of the potential complications and use them judiciously, especially when children are around.

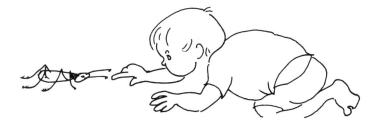

Walker Injuries

*N*ine-month-old Pedro scuttled across the dining room in his walker. He stepped on a few toys, as he could not see where he was going, then accelerated in the walker, which went under the dining table, hit his head hard against the table, and passed out for a few seconds. Pedro's mother panicked and rushed him to the emergency room.

Each year, parents in this country buy more than 3 million walkers. Parents feel that the walkers are useful in promoting mobility, keeping infants quiet and happy, and providing some exercise. Some believe that walkers offer their infants safety as well. Many of these beliefs are wrong.

About 12 to 40 percent of infants in walkers sustain injuries. Many more injuries occur that need no medical attention. The annual incidence of walker injuries resulting in visits to an emergency room is about 8.9 per 1000 children less than 1 year of age. One fourth of these injuries are severe, namely, fractures and closed head injuries. In one study, 10 percent of all walker injuries were found to be skull fractures. Severe injuries have almost always occurred from falls down the stairs in a walker.

Burns and poisonings have also occurred because the infant is mobile and can reach for the source of the fire or poison easily. Children in walkers can propel themselves at a speed of three feet per second, accumulating a lot of kinetic energy, so a supervising adult has very little time to prevent an accident. In addition, pinch injuries to fingers and toes have occurred because of the walkers.

In addition to injuries, walkers cause harm by delaying a child's motor and mental development. Siegel and Burton in 1999 studied 109 infants between the ages of 6 and 15 months, with or without walker experience. They found that children who used walkers sat, crawled, and walked later than children who did not use the walkers. Also, children using walkers scored lower in the mental and motor development tests. The greatest negative influence was noticed in mental development in the 6-to-9 months age period. In some infants the deleterious effect of walker use was measurable as long as 10 months after the initial use.

Why is it so? Modern walkers have large opaque trays and small leg openings designed to prevent tripping. The infant cannot see his or her legs and feet. Visual feedback about the body position and limb movement is necessary for the timely development of motor milestones. When this feedback is lacking, the infant experiences motor developmental delays.

Considering the risk of severe injuries and delayed motor and mental development, the American Academy of Pediatrics has recommended a ban on selling mobile walkers. It is a good idea not to buy them, but we still see them in shops and people are still buying them. Meanwhile, public education, adult supervision during walker use, and barriers such as stair-gates should reduce walker injuries.

Pedro's head injury was not serious; he was sent home from the ER with head injury instructions. When I checked him the next day, he was doing well.

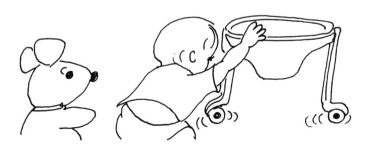

Dangerous Waters, Even at Home

Eight-year-old May went on a school trip to a public swimming pool. Even though the teachers were vigilant, May wandered away unnoticed. There were many children swimming, and no one knew when May entered the pool; someone suddenly noticed that she was lying unconscious in the bottom of the pool, and a lifeguard pulled her out immediately. She was given CPR and rushed to the emergency room by ambulance.

In children, drowning is the second most common cause of death, motor vehicular accidents being number one. Approximately 150,000 persons drown each year, amounting to one person every 3.5 minutes. Children are particularly at risk. About 8,000 children drown every year in the United States. Pediatric drowning constitutes 7 percent of deaths in children who are less than one year of age, 19 percent in 1 to 4 year olds, and 12 to14 percent in older children.

Residential swimming pools are the most common drowning site for young children; 90 percent are children less than five years old. In California, there were 3,000 annual ER visits because of this; 80 percent of these children needed hospitalization at least for a day, costing 5.2 million dollars annually.

Bathtubs account for 86 percent of drowning deaths in children between the ages of 7 and 15 months. Hot tubs and spas are also dangerous because many have suction devices in which clothing, hair, or body parts get caught. Children can also drown in buckets, toilets, washing machines, and sinks with water. Children aged 7 to 15 months account for 88 percent of bucket deaths. Children fall headfirst into the buckets and cannot right themselves. In all these incidents, brief lapses in supervision (less than five minutes) are responsible for the drownings.

Older children and adolescents usually drown in lakes, ponds, and rivers. One fifth of these drowning accidents involve boats. In half of them alcohol and drugs are the culprits.

What are the complications of drowning? Damage to various organs due to the lack of oxygen, aspiration pneumonia, fluid and electrolyte disturbances, hypothermia, and death are the major outcomes. About 80 percent of children in water submersions survive and 92 percent of the survivors recover completely. From 13 to 35 percent of children admitted to intensive care units die, and 7 to 27 percent survive with severe brain damage.

How can one prevent drowning accidents? Parents and caregivers should be aware of how easy it is for children to drown in less than five minutes and that water anywhere, even in small quantities, poses a drowning risk. About 75 percent of the residential swimming pools are inadequately fenced and proper fencing should be done keeping in mind that some children can climb over it easily.

At least one person in the house should know CPR; about 42 percent of the children who drowned were not given CPR until the ambulance staff arrived. Buckets with water or detergents should not be left unattended. Toilet covers and bathroom doors should be kept closed always.

Swimming lessons for two to four-year-olds won't guarantee protection from drowning. While swimming in lakes and rivers, children and adolescents should wear life vests and never swim alone.

Adults should also avoid alcohol and drugs while in the water. These simple rules will save lives.

With supportive care, May recovered in the emergency room. She was kept for a day in the hospital and discharged the next day and did well.

Mini-Scooters? Major Injuries!

*J*oseph, 11 years old, took a ride on a mini-scooter, just to try it out. It looked simple and fun. In a few seconds, the scooter hit an uneven spot on the sidewalk; Joseph lost his balance. As he fell down, he tried to protect his head with his hands. When he got up, he felt a terrible pain over his left little finger and palm. The hand began to swell.

"Mom, I think I broke my hand," Joseph announced as he entered the house.

"You're kidding! You just walked out! I don't believe you," his mother replied.

But it was true—Joseph had broken one of the bones in his palm, which was confirmed by an X ray. I had to send him to the Emergency Room and then to an orthopedic specialist to take care of his fracture.

Mini-scooters have very small wheels that get stuck easily in crevices on the road, but they are the "in" thing nowadays. Every kid on my block has one. Even though statistics are not available for mini-scooter injuries, they are likely to be similar to those caused by skateboards and roller skates as all of them have small wheels. There is plenty of data available on skateboard and roller skate injuries.

A study conducted by the Emergency Department of George Washington University showed similar injuries occurring with in-line skates, skateboards, and roller skates. Minor injuries included bruises, sprains, and lacerations. However, about 43 percent of the injuries were serious, involving a fracture of the hand or forearm. One third of the fractures involved bad alignment of the broken bones. Head, knee, and ankle injuries also occurred, but less frequently. More injuries and fractures were noticed in children not wearing any protective devices.

Most of the injuries occurred as the child skated on the street or sidewalk. The child was skating too fast in 35 percent of the accidents, struck an object on the pavement 20 percent of the time, and in 19 percent of the cases was either unable to stop or hit a motor vehicle. Even though parents and adolescents were aware of the potentiality for accidents, 75 percent of the skaters did not use any protective devices.

Supervise your children and make sure they wear protective gear such as a helmet, elbow and wrist guards, and kneepads. Advise them not to skate on streets and near driveways, and watch for traffic. Check their immunizations and make sure that their tetanus shots are current. As always, an ounce of prevention is better than a ton of cure.

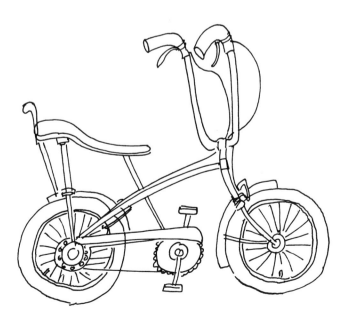

This Should Never Happen

*H*eather, 11 years old, came to my office with her foster mother. Heather had multiple problems. Even though her height and weight were normal, her motor and mental development lagged, and she rocked back and forth while standing. She had an obsessive behavior of touching her ears, chin, and tongue repeatedly; she would also close an eye and press it hard with her fingers. She was in a special class in fourth grade. While doing mathematics, she would pause often and go through the behaviors mentioned earlier. If she did something wrong, she would not accept it, but would blame others. Moreover, Heather's attention span was short; she had attention deficit disorder and was on a medication to alleviate the symptoms.

When I examined Heather, she was cooperative, but exhibited the ritualistic behavior. She had strabismus and wore corrective glasses; she also had a moderate hearing loss. Examination of the heart revealed a loud murmur that, I later came to know, was due to the narrowing of the pulmonary artery, the major blood vessel that carries deoxygenated blood to the lungs; the narrowed artery creates a condition known as "pulmonary stenosis". I noticed thickening of the skin of the wrist due to constant rubbing of the arms. Heather's feet were flat and she had difficulty hopping.

I continued her medications for attention deficit disorder, and monitored her blood counts and liver functions because these could be affected by the treatment. Further, her heart condition made it necessary for her to be given antibiotics even for small procedures such as dental cleaning, or minor operations.

Why did Heather develop eye problems, pulmonary stenosis, flat feet, odd behaviors, and attention deficiency? She was suffering from the damage done to her by German measles or rubella, while she was still in her mother's womb. Children who have been affected by rubella in this manner exhibit complex signs and symptoms that are called "Congenital Rubella Syndrome".

Even though the rubella virus causes only a mild disease in pregnant mothers, it may play havoc with the fetus. The consequences of fetal rubella infection are varied and unpredictable. Spontaneous abortion, still birth, and live birth with congenital malformations have all been documented in medical literature; so has the birth of normal infants. Some unfortunate infants suffer from cardiac defects, hearing loss, eye problems like cataracts and glaucoma, abnormal behaviors, attention deficit, and neurological defects. In addition they may develop endocrine problems, such as insulin dependent diabetes mellitus.

I never saw Heather's mother. She probably never got immunized against rubella and had the disease in the first few weeks when she was carrying Heather.

I urge adolescent girls to check their immunizations. If a combination vaccine against measles, mumps, and rubella called MMR has not been given or only one MMR has been given so far, teenagers should contact their doctors to get the immunizations updated. What Heather had is preventable and should never happen to your child.

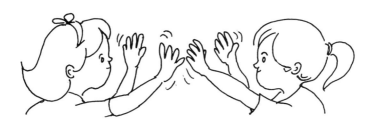

Cholesterol in Children

en-year-old Greg came to my office for a physical examination. Even though he was 4 feet 10 inches tall, a normal height for his age, he weighed 140 pounds, which was well above the normal range. His cholesterol was slightly elevated, including the low-density lipoprotein (LDL) that is commonly called the "bad cholesterol". All this was because he especially loved to eat potato chips and other fried snacks, and his favorite breakfast was scrambled eggs. An ounce of yolk, present in approximately two eggs, has 10 grams of fat and 480 milligrams of cholesterol. Egg yolk has more than 10 times the amount of cholesterol contained in an equal amount of beef or pork. An ounce of potato chips has 10 grams of fat, but no cholesterol.

Adult heart disease has its early roots in childhood eating habits. High cholesterol levels measured in young adults in their twenties correlated with coronary heart disease (CHD) that developed 30 or 40 years later. Increased cholesterol and LDL levels cause atherosclerosis, a hardening of the arteries in the heart, brain, and other organs that leads to a blockage of the blood vessels, causing heart attacks and strokes.

Who made the connection between cholesterol and atherosclerosis? In the history of medicine, some important discoveries often go unnoticed. Nikolai Amchkov, a Russian physician, was the first to notice that cholesterol caused atherosclerosis. Earlier, Ignatowski, a Russian clinician, had fed eggs and milk to rabbits, and noticed hardening of their arteries. He believed, erroneously, that milk and egg proteins caused atherosclerosis.

N.W. Stuckey, Amchkov's colleague, devised an elegant experiment. He fed muscle proteins to one group of rabbits, egg whites to a second group, and egg yolk to a third group. The rabbits who consumed the egg yolk developed atherosclerosis. Another one of Amchkov's colleagues examined the hardened vessels and found fat-like droplets that, under polarized light, could be identified as cholesterol. Then, the scientists fed pure cholesterol to rabbits, who eventually developed atherosclerosis. It didn't mean that the same would happen in humans, but the experiment showed a cause and effect superbly. In 1912, Amchkov was awarded a traveling fellowship. However, his pioneering work was not fully recognized.

In 1950, J. W. Gofman, using a high-speed centrifuge that rotated 40,000 times a minute, separated cholesterol into high density (HDL) and low-density (LDL) fractions. After many studies, the researchers concluded that elevated LDL levels also caused atherosclerosis. About the same time, Dr. Kinsell in Alameda, California, discovered that eating vegetables and avoiding animal fats lowered the cholesterol. The hospital administrator did not appreciate his pioneering work and cut off his admission bed allocations for research. As the hospital was unknown, he could not get grants to conduct his research. In desperation, he committed suicide. The right person in the wrong place!

Based on what we know now, I advised Greg to exercise regularly. I told his mother not to buy potato chips, and to feed Gregg only egg whites. When he lost a few pounds, his cholesterol and LDL came down, and he greeted me with a broad smile.

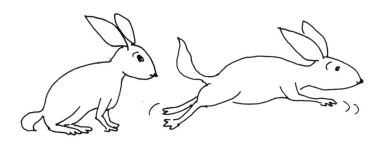

More Precious Than Gold!

Elizabeth came to me with her mother, Mrs. Walters, for a health check up. Then just eighteen months old, she was cute and chubby, weighing six pounds more than girls her age. Mrs. Walters commented that Elizabeth was irritable and seemed to have a poor appetite, except for milk. Occasionally she had seen Elizabeth eat earth and ice chips.

"Why does she do that?" Mrs. Walters asked me.

"Eating earth, ice, etc., is called pica. Some children with anemia do that. By the way, how much milk does Elizabeth consume daily?" I asked.

"About ten bottles."

That came to five pints of milk a day. Elizabeth was overweight because she consumed excessive amounts of milk. Since such children often are anemic, I ran a few tests on her.

Anemia is defined as a lower than normal quantity of hemoglobin or red blood cells. Elizabeth's hemoglobin, the oxygen-carrying pigment, was at seven grams percent. Normally at her age she should have had at least eleven grams. Her serum iron was low and the total quantity of iron in her body was low. Traces of blood were found in her stools. By appropriate tests, major causes of blood loss from her intestines were eliminated. Because she had pica, I did a blood lead level, but there was no significant amount of lead. The tests showed that Elizabeth had an anemia due to iron deficiency.

How did this happen? Cow's milk has very little iron and what exists is poorly absorbed. In some children, milk protein sensitizes the intestines and causes microscopic bleeding which enhances the anemia. Moreover, Elizabeth wasn't eating solid foods containing iron. All these factors caused iron deficiency anemia.

Children with moderate iron deficiency have anemia, irritability, and poor appetite. Even without anemia, some children who have iron deficiency have a short attention span, lack alertness, experience difficulty in learning, and perform poorly at school. That's why it is important to recognize iron deficiency and treat it promptly.

I explained all this to Mrs. Walters and instructed her not to give Elizabeth more than two cups of milk a day. Elizabeth could also have more solid foods rich in iron such as iron fortified grains and cereals, meat, egg yolks, tomatoes, and green and yellow vegetables. I also started Elizabeth on ferrous sulfate drops. In a couple of days, Elizabeth was less irritable and in two months her hemoglobin value was normal.

Our bodies need iron, not just for the manufacture of hemoglobin, but to form a muscle protein called myoglobin. Iron is part of many enzymes in our body, including those in the nervous system, that help transport oxygen. Because iron is involved in such crucial functions, our body conserves iron like a miser. Only ten percent of a body's total iron stores are lost in a year. Gold may seem precious to us human beings, but for the human body iron is more precious than gold!

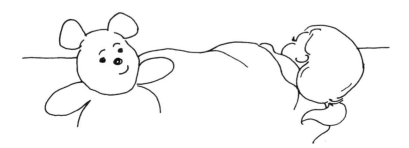

Elegant Solution to a Bitter Problem

iffany had an ear infection. I prescribed an antibiotic, and advised her mother to give her the medication regularly. When I checked Tiffany after a week, her ear infection was still present.

There are several reasons why an ear infection could persist in a child who is on antibiotics. The infection could be due to a virus, and antibiotics are ineffective against viruses; or the infection could be bacterial, and the bacteria may have developed a resistance to the antibiotic; or the child may not have been given the antibiotics properly, with either a smaller dose being given or several doses being missed. I explained all these possibilities to Tiffany's mother.

"Doc, the antibiotic that you gave tastes terrible," Tiffany's mother said. "My baby spits it up. If I force her to take it, she throws up. To tell you frankly, I stopped giving it after a couple of days. Sorry!"

It is true that some medications taste terrible. Children have taste preferences and some hate certain antibiotics and will not take them. Full-term newborns and even premature infants have the ability to detect sweets and reject bitter solutions. Perhaps, long ago, this quality had a survival advantage, favoring animals who consumed high-energy, vitamin-mineral-rich fruit and vegetable diets, while avoiding bitter poisonous fruits and plants. If the medications leave a bitter aftertaste children will not take them. Traditionally, parents mix medications with various foods like fruit yogurt, honey, applesauce, juices, etc. But which food is good at masking the bitter taste?

Enter Dr. Schwartz. He and his colleagues conducted a study

to determine the masking quality of various food items for bitter taste. They tested tropical fruit punch, grape juice, applesauce, strawberry syrup, and nonfat chocolate syrup on a total of 107 children, ranging in age from 3 to 8 years. The study was designed in such a way that subjective errors were eliminated. At the end of the study, Dr. Schwartz concluded that chocolate syrup given immediately after a bitter-tasting antibiotic masked the unpleasant taste the best.

I told Tiffany's mother to try nonfat chocolate syrup. Tiffany liked it and finished the antibiotic without a problem. Milton Hershey would be very happy to know that the chocolate he popularized 100 years ago is helping children to swallow unpalatable antibiotics today!

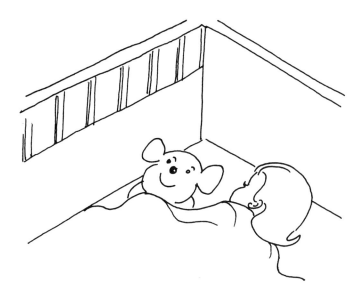

Today's Good Nutrition Makes Tomorrow's Strong Bones

*S*tacy was 16 years old, weighed 105 pounds, and was five feet six inches tall. Thin and lovely as a model, she was full of energy, and exercised regularly. Obsessed about gaining too much weight, she watched her diet, avoiding any foods containing fat, including cheese. She consumed about a cup of skim milk and fat-free yogurt a day. She ate meat sparingly. However, she ate a lot of vegetables and fruits, and avoided nuts.

During one of Stacy's office visits, I told her that she was not getting enough fat in her foods. I pointed out that fats are essential for the integrity of cell membranes and nuclei of cells, and they form a protective coating around nerves, blood vessels, and organs. Fats also need to be consumed for the proper absorption of such vitamins as A, D, E, and K. At least 20 to 30 percent of calories must be from fats. Moreover, because she was taking minimal amounts of milk and milk products, she was not getting enough calcium.

"I eat lots of vegetables, Dr. Rao," Stacy said. "Don't I get enough calcium?"

I was not very familiar with the calcium content of foods, so I promptly read up on it. What we eat now has a profound effect on our health later in life. Consuming lesser amounts of calcium can later lead to brittle bones, a condition called osteoporosis. As a nation, we spend 13.8 billion dollars a year treating fractures due to osteoporosis. Once osteoporosis develops there is no cure; the good news is that it is preventable.

Rapid gain in bone mass happens during childhood, and between 11 and 14 years of age in girls. Weight-bearing physical activity also increases bone mass, provided the adolescent consumes enough calcium in food. For children 9 to 18 years of age, the recommended daily allowance of calcium is 1,300 milligrams.

Can foods alone provide this amount of calcium? To get 1,300 milligrams of calcium, a teenager should take approximately four cups of milk or yogurt a day, or four cups of macaroni and cheese. Other foods having the same quantity of calcium individually are 6.5 ounces of cheese; four slices of cheese pizza; four cups of calcium enriched orange juice; three cups of tofu; eight cups of broccoli; 28 cups of beans; or 32 cups of spinach. We can be sure Stacy was not eating eight cups of broccoli or 32 cups of spinach daily!

Many teenagers' diets are deficient in calcium. On an average, a teenager's food contains 790 milligrams of calcium, which is far below the daily requirements. If she or he does not take milk or milk products, the calcium intake is further diminished. Moreover, a high salt intake minimizes calcium absorption. Thus, teenagers eating hamburgers and potato chips that have high amounts of salt are prone to calcium deficiency. Diminished bone mass leads to osteoporosis later in life.

I told Stacy to add more dairy products to her diet. Because Stacy would still receive only some 790 milligrams of calcium, I advised her to drink a couple of cups of calcium-fortified orange juice daily, or have one TUMS tablet twice daily with food.

"Take good care of your bones now, and they'll take care of you in your old age," I said.

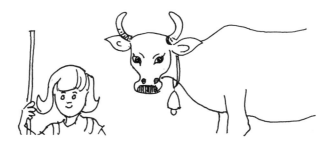

Are We Feeding Our Children Right?

One child in four in my practice is overweight. The incidence of diabetes has become an epidemic among children because of obesity. Are we not feeding our children properly?

Following the 1992 recommendations of the U. S. Department of Agriculture, doctors and nutritionists have been advising people to consume 6-11 daily servings of bread, cereal, rice, and pasta daily, and to eat fatty foods, oils, and sweets sparingly. Of course they recommend other items such as fruits, and vegetables such as potatoes, broccoli, carrots, grapes, apples, and bananas. Meat, fish, poultry, milk and other foods are also to be consumed. Basically, they have been telling us to avoid fatty foods, and to eat plenty of carbohydrates.

Is this sound advice? Are carbohydrates good and fats that bad?

Parents need to be aware of what happens when one consumes a large quantity of refined pasta, white bread, or baked potato. The body very quickly converts these foods into glucose, the blood glucose level rises, and this prompts an immediate release of a large quantity of insulin. The blood glucose level then falls, sometimes even below normal; the child feels hungry again and eats some more, which eventually leads to obesity. The incidence of diabetes mellitus is higher in children and adults who consume large quantities of refined carbohydrates.

Moreover, high blood glucose and increased insulin raises triglycerides and lowers the good cholesterol, setting the stage for later heart attacks and strokes.

Now the facts about fats. Saturated fats in food such as butter and red meat are bad because they raise the bad cholesterol (LDL) level in the blood. A higher level of LDL is well correlated with an increased risk of heart attacks and strokes. Another class of fats called trans-unsaturated fatty acids (trans fats) are as bad as saturated fats. The trans fats are produced by frying or by hydrogenation of vegetable oils, and are present in margarine, fried foods, and some baked foods. They too raise the LDL and triglycerides, and hence are detrimental to our health.

Fortunately, certain other fats are beneficial to our health. Fish, fish oils, and walnuts contain omega-3 fatty acids that prevent heart disease. Olive oil has mono-unsaturated fatty acids, and peanuts and peanut oil have poly-unsaturated fatty acids that prevent heart attacks and strokes. Moreover, eating nuts satisfies one's appetite and so the individual eats less.

Epidemiological studies prove the beneficial effects of eating more of the foods that contain unsaturated fatty acids. People in Eastern Finland eat a diet that contains 38 percent of fat from milk, butter, etc., that is mostly of a saturated variety. The incidence of heart disease in that area is 3,000 per 10,000 population over a period of ten years. In comparison, people on the island of Crete consume a diet that contains 40 percent of fat, mostly of the unsaturated type, from olives and olive oil, fish, etc. Even though the consumption of fat is about the same, the incidence of heart disease in Crete is only 200 per 10,000 population, far less than in East Finland; the quality of the fat being consumed obviously accounts for the difference. Remarkably, the low incidence of heart problems in Crete is even better than in Japan; although the Japanese diet contains only 10 percent of fat, the incidence of heart disease is 500 per 10,000 men, over a period of ten years.

What do nutrition pundits recommend now?

First of all, get everyone in the family off the couch and into exercise. Control your weight—it is good for your heart and your health. Don't be lured into buying and serving "combo meals", and avoid "all you can eat" deals in restaurants. Instead, eat smaller portions. Eat more of foods such as fish, items prepared with vegetable oils, and nuts, all of which contain mono and poly-unsaturated fatty acids. However, as oils and nuts have twice the calories of carbohydrates and proteins, eat them in moderation.

Avoid saturated fats and trans fat foods. Choose unrefined carbohydrates such as whole wheat bread, oatmeal, and brown rice. Of course, eat vegetables and fruits in plenty. Limit taking red meat; instead, consume poultry. Such a modified diet has resulted in a significant reduction of heart disease, up to 30 percent for women and 40 percent for men.

Get your family to eat smart, and live long!

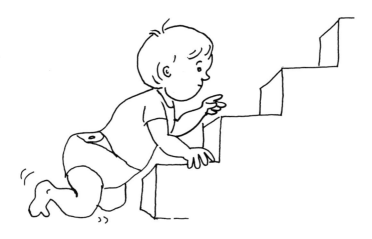

An Apple a Day? Yes, With the Skin!

My colleague was biting an apple vigorously as I entered the physicians' room.

"Just to keep the doctor away," she said, smiling, and bit off another chunk of it.

Is the saying true? Are apples indeed better, or are they just like any other fruit, supplying vitamin C, minerals, and fiber? Vitamin C is an antioxidant and protects against cell damage that leads to aging. Then, why not just take the vitamin C as a pill? Are there any other benefits in the one-a-day apple? Did our forefathers know something that we did not appreciate? I pondered over these questions.

Recently, Marian Eberhardt and colleagues at Cornell University performed several elegant experiments on extracts of Red Delicious apples. They measured the antioxidant properties of the extracts and came up with numbers depicting the degree of antioxidant activity. They found that the antioxidant effect of extracts of an apple with skin was greater than the effect noticed from extracts of the fruit without the skin. Moreover, 100 grams of extract of apple-with-skin had only 5.7 milligrams of vitamin C, but the antioxidant activity was equivalent to 1500 mgs of vitamin C. They surmised that most of the protective effect of the extract was due to chemicals other than vitamin C, such as flavonoids, phenolics, and quercetin glycosides.

The scientists next incubated these extracts with colon cancer cells of the Caco-2 cell line, and found that apple extracts inhibited the growth of the cancer cells. The extract of apple with skin had a one-and-a-half times greater inhibiting effect on the proliferation of cancer cells than the extract of apple pulp alone.

Then the investigators tested the extracts against the growth of human liver cancer cells. Again they noticed inhibition in the growth of the cells, more so with the apple-with-skin extracts.

It seems that the natural chemicals in the apple such as flavonoids and phenolic acids have a strong inhibitory effect on the proliferation of some cancers. Interestingly, the skin of the apple has more phenolics than the pulp. Glycosides are found only in the skin. So it makes a lot of sense to grab an apple and eat it with its skin on, just to keep the doctors away!

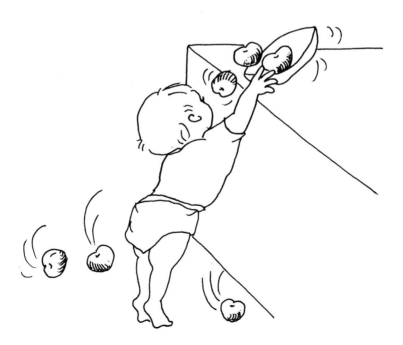

Is Chocolate Good for Your Child?

Chocolate hearts and Hershey Kisses left over from Valentine's Day sat on my table for days, tempting me to reach out and taste them. Though my mouth watered, the quantity of fat and sugar in each piece dampened my desire to savor them. Still, I wondered whether chocolates contained anything that would be beneficial to my health. Since children love chocolates, too, I decided to investigate.

Recent studies have shown that chocolate contains flavanols—-chemicals similar to those found in tea, fruits, and red wine—that are helpful to our cardiovascular health. Cocoa flavanols are found to cause dilatation of blood vessels, reduce damage to them, and delay blood clotting.

In laboratories, cocoa flavanols are found to produce vascular dilatation by increasing nitric oxide, which relaxes the smooth muscle in blood vessels. Dr. Carl Keen, professor of nutrition at the University of California at Davis, has studied populations that consume foods rich in flavanols. One such population with a high intake of cocoa flavanols in their diet has low blood pressure, which is beneficial.

Scientists from the Royal Melbourne Institute of Technology in Australia studied the long-term effects of cocoa on platelet function. Platelets are small particles in the blood that are essential for clotting. They help to stop bleeding from a cut. However, under certain conditions, platelets adhere and form clots inside a blood vessel, which may lead to a heart attack or a stroke. In a preliminary study, the scientists evaluated 32 healthy individuals by offering them 234 mgs. of cocoa flavanols to consume daily. After four weeks, platelet aggregation and clotting were significantly lower in the group that consumed cocoa flavanols, compared to the group that consumed the placebo.

Flavanols have a good effect on cholesterol as well. Low-density lipoprotein (LDL) is known as bad cholesterol; in elevated levels it damages blood vessels, promotes clot formation, and predisposes one to heart attacks and strokes. However, for LDL to have a detrimental effect on blood vessels, it must first be oxidized, and that is where chocolate can help. Preliminary laboratory experiments at UC Davis have shown that cocoa flavanols inhibit the oxidation of LDL and so prevent blood vessel damage. In human trials, lipid oxidation products decreased in the circulation, and antioxidant effects increased, within two hours of chocolate having been eaten.

But is the fat content in chocolate not harmful? Fats in chocolate are saturated fatty acids, namely, stearic and palmitic acids; though, generally speaking, saturated fat is bad for health, chocolate also contains oleic acid, which is an unsaturated fatty acid. Also, it was discovered that the stearic acid in chocolate did not affect LDL and HDL levels in men, though it did lower the HDL level in women. More research is needed.

Be aware that not all chocolates are created equal; many flavanols are destroyed during the processing of cocoa beans. However, Mars Incorporated has a proprietary method of cocoa processing that preserves flavanols.

I pondered over these studies. Even though the final word is not out, it seems that chocolate is good for the blood vessels and prevents clot formation.

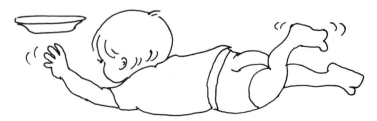

Coffee Pros and Cons

People have been drinking coffee for at least 3,000 years. On a foggy day, there is nothing more joyous than waking up to a cup of freshly brewed coffee; my own family loves the brew and its alluring aromas and unique flavors. Coffee is the world's most popular beverage and about 1.1 billion cups are consumed every day worldwide. In the United States, 52 percent of adults drink coffee everyday; on average, Americans consume 3.3 cups of coffee a day.

Coffee, in addition to having caffeine, has more than 800 chemicals in it. Are there any ill effects to drinking coffee? Is it good for health?

Let me first state the negatives. Excessive coffee drinking may irritate the stomach and aggravate an ulcer. Even though there are no conclusive studies at this moment, coffee may increase the risk of a heart attack by causing a stress reaction. Scientists from Duke University Medical Center found that four to five cups of coffee in the morning raise blood pressure and

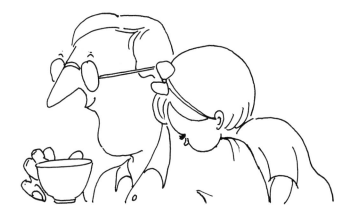

increase the level of adrenaline by 32 percent. In other words, coffee adds to the day-to-day stress that may do harm in the long run. However, doctors from the British Nutrition Institute say that there is not enough evidence that coffee increases the risk of a heart attack.

By general agreement, young children are seldom offered coffee. Pregnant women may drink coffee in moderation, limiting intake to one or two cups a day; drinking more than 4 cups of coffee a day will double the risk of miscarriage. Of course, expectant mothers who drink coffee should then watch for other items that have caffeine, such as sodas and chocolate, because caffeine can cause seizures in the newborn child.

Still on the negative side, Finnish researchers have discovered that coffee drinking is associated with the presence of rheumatoid factor, an antibody found in people with rheumatoid arthritis. Perhaps this is one more environmental factor that can precipitate the arthritis.

Now, what are the benefits of coffee? Coffee has a chemical called dihydrocaffeic acid, which is an antioxidant. It is well known that antioxidants help us to live longer in a healthier state.

Coffee is a stimulant and increases athletic performance. But it also has a positive effect on thinking. In the geriatric population, cognitive performance was better with coffee, especially in women older than 80 years. So, can coffee prevent Alzheimer's disease? Scientists of the Faculty of Medicine in Lisbon have found that old people who did not have Alzheimer's disease, as compared to people who had the disease, were drinking over two cups of brewed coffee a day. Maybe we should serve more coffee in nursing homes!

Epidemiological studies show a decreased incidence of colorectal cancer in regular coffee drinkers. A couple of chemicals in coffee, cafestol and kahwol, have proven to have anticancer properties in animals. Coffee has a laxative effect; perhaps by moving the bowels regularly, coffee may prevent cancer-causing chemicals from irritating the bowel, thus reducing the occurrence of cancer.

By analyzing the health and lifestyle database of 17,000 Dutch individuals, scientists found that people who drank seven or more cups of coffee a day had a 50 percent lesser incidence of Type 2 diabetes, so coffee may protect against Type 2 diabetes as well. But seven or more cups is a lot of coffee to drink!

So how many cups of coffee should you drink a day? If you don't have a medical problem, scientists say that two to four cups a day will not harm, but in fact may do you some good. You may not remember all the pros and cons I mentioned, but if you and your teenagers are offered a cup of good coffee, go ahead and just enjoy it!

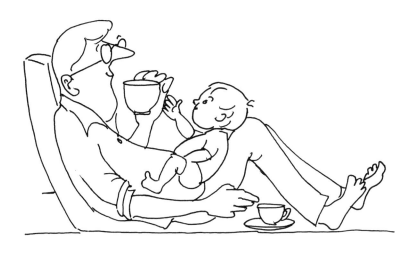

Good Bacteria, Bad Bacteria

amela, 15 months old, was brought to my office for an ear infection. I gave her an antibiotic. Three days later she came back with profuse diarrhea and a diaper rash. Why did Pamela develop severe diarrhea after starting the antibiotic? Why did she develop the diaper rash? To understand this, we need to know a little about the helpful bacteria that live both inside us and on our skin.

Bacteria and fungi are everywhere. Normally, about 12 kinds of bacteria live on the skin, eight more varieties live in the small gut, and another 23 species in the large intestine. The mouth is even worse; 30 strains of germs inhabit the oral cavity. Most of these bacteria are helpful to a normal person. They constantly stimulate the immune system and keep it primed; the good bacteria also prevent the bad ones from adhering to the gut wall by producing hydrogen peroxide and other chemicals that are inimical to them. For example, a germ called *helicobacter pylori* causes stomach ulcers. The good bacteria are known to displace the helicobacter and thus help to heal the ulcer.

What are these good bacteria? There are many. *Lactobacillus* GG and *lactobacillus acidophilus* are two examples. These harmless bacteria live in the gut in large numbers and occupy the surface of the gut mucous membrane, thus preventing the bad ones from getting a foothold; or rather, I should say, a flagellum hold.

Lactobacillus GG and Lactobacillus acidophilus are also present in large amounts in yogurt, but one has to read the label carefully to note the presence of live cultures of such bacteria. Capsules are also available in health food stores. Such biological substances are called "probiotics." In randomized controlled studies, lactobacilli were found to be beneficial in reducing high blood pressure, cholesterol, allergy, and asthma, and also decreased the severity of symptoms of an intestinal ailment called Crohn's disease. In children, the lactobacilli reduced the incidence of rotavirus induced diarrhea and diaper rash.

In one study, children in daycare who drank an average of 260 ml of milk containing lactobacillus GG daily for seven months had fewer ear infections, lower respiratory infections, and less sinusitis than those who drank unsupplemented milk. In another study, ingesting the lactobacillus reduced the risk of eczema by 50 percent when given to non-breast-fed infants for the first six months after birth.

Swedish scientists did an interesting study. They sprayed alpha-hemolytic streptococci in the noses of volunteers. These bacteria are harmless. When they colonized in the nose and mouth, they effectively prevented the growth of disease-causing bacteria. Children who took part had fewer ear infections.

Would you believe that pinworms have a protective effect on your intestines? Over the past 30 years, pinworm infections have declined in developed nations, and there has been a concomitant increase in inflammatory bowel disease. The disease, which causes abdominal pain and diarrhea, is uncommon in developing countries where there are plenty of pinworm infections. In a study from the University of Iowa, people suffering from inflammatory bowel disease were infected with harmless intestinal worms. Seven out of eight patients' symptoms improved immediately.

When Pamela took the antibiotic for an ear infection, it destroyed the good bacteria in her intestines. Pamela had diarrhea either because of an invasion by another disease-causing bacterium or irritation by the antibiotic. The diaper rash was due to a skin infection by a fungus called *candida albicans*. The antibiotic killed the helpful bacteria setting the stage for the fungus to invade.

Probiotics are being increasingly used in preventing some diseases. I gave Pamela an antifungal ointment for her diaper rash and told Pamela's mother to give her yogurt with active cultures of lactobacillus acidophilus and other lactobacilli, in the hope that these beneficial bacilli would replace the bad ones in her gut. Pamela recovered fast.

A constant war is being waged between good and bad bacteria for premium real estate inside and outside of our bodies. Maintaining good health ultimately depends on a fine balance between the good germs and the bad.

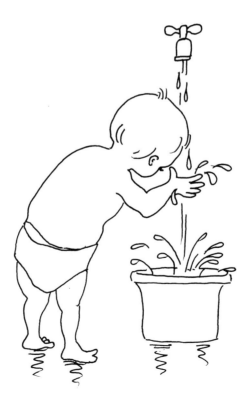

What You Eat Is
What You'll Become

In his popular television show some years ago, the comedian Flip Wilson, dressed up as a buxom young woman, had a favorite punch line, "What you see is what you get!" I would prefer to say, "What you eat is what you'll become!" We are learning that intelligently selecting foods we eat will prevent quite a few diseases and prolong your life. I will briefly write about some of the diseases that are preventable by consuming the proper foods.

Coronary Heart Disease (CHD): Eating butter, lard, hydrogenated oils and other saturated fats leads to an increase in low density lipoprotein (LDL), called bad cholesterol. It is aptly named "bad" because increased levels of LDL lead to a hardening of the arteries (atherosclerosis) that leads to strokes and heart attacks. High density lipoprotein (HDL), also known as good cholesterol, prevents atherosclerosis.

How do you help lower your child's LDL? Avoid serving your family the foods mentioned earlier. Use small amounts of olive oil to cook. Steam, bake, or broil. Don't fry. As for yourself, if you drink, take moderate amounts of red wine if your doctor approves it. Red wine increases the HDL. Alcohol is a double-edged weapon, though. It may cause a stomach ulcer, liver damage, pancreatic inflammation, and other complications. As an alternative, you can drink red grape juice, which has about ¼ the effect of red wine.

Another simple way to lower the LDL and increase the HDL is to get the family off the couch. Exercise, walk, jog, cycle a mile or two a day, or play active games together as a family; an active child has a far better chance of staying a healthy child.

Eating fish at least twice a week, or taking fish oils, will protect against future sudden death due to arrhythmias during a heart attack. Also, fish oils lower high blood pressure, and may help improve psoriasis and rheumatoid arthritis. In certain kidney diseases, fish oil reduces damage to that organ.

LDL needs to be oxidized before it can damage a blood vessel. Vitamins like C and E and beta-carotene prevent the oxidation of LDL. They are called antioxidants. In one study, vitamin E supplementation reduced the incidence of myocardial infarction. Think of bright colors to pep up the family meals! Red tomatoes, green bell peppers, orange carrots and so on. Citrus fruits and tomatoes are rich in vitamin C. Legumes, vegetables, and vegetable oils are rich in vitamin E. Beta-carotene is found in carrots and vegetables. Eat them in abundance.

Tea has plenty of antioxidants. Drinking black or green tea prevents heart attacks and strokes. Coffee, even though it has antioxidants, may irritate and aggravate stomach ulcers. However, coffee can reduce the risk of contracting Alzheimer's disease and protects against tooth decay.

An amino acid called homocysteine is elevated in people who are prone to coronary heart disease. Folic acid lowers the homocysteine level. So eat foods such as legumes and fresh green leafy vegetables that are rich in folic acid, which can lower homocysteine.

Cancer: We are constantly exposed to many cancer-causing substances. As a result, free radicals are liberated and mutations occur in the cells. Normally these radicals are removed and the damage is repaired promptly. Folic acid and Vitamins C and E improve the capacity of cells to repair the damage. Hence plan to eat the foods mentioned earlier that are rich in folic acid, and in vitamins C and E. Do not take mega-doses of vitamins unless approved by your doctor. To give you an example, vitamin C in a small dose acts as an antioxidant, but in large doses may increase oxidation and cause more harm.

Vegetables such as broccoli, cabbage, and kale have a chemical called sulforaphane that is protective against cancer. Many fruits have cancer-fighting compounds in them. Raspberries have ellagic acid that prevents tumor growth. Cherries are full of perillyl alcohol, which seems to offer protection against breast, colon, and prostate cancers. The skin of an apple has plenty of fiber and lots of cancer-protective antioxidants. So eat plenty of fruits and vegetables.

Obesity and excessive alcohol consumption predispose a person to breast cancer development. Eating less fat and consuming more fiber-containing foods with adequate calcium and folic acid helps to prevent colorectal cancer. Take heed and modify your food habits.

High Blood Pressure: Weight control and exercise reduce blood pressure. Adequate calcium intake (non-fat milk, enriched juices) and eating fish or fish oils will also bring down high blood pressure to some extent.

Osteoporosis: Inadequate calcium intake during childhood leads to a decrease in bone-mass that may cause osteoporosis later in life. So give your children calcium fortified breads, juices, and dairy products, keeping an eye on their fat content. You too should eat these food items.

Constipation: Chronic constipation may cause intestinal diverticular disease. Make sure you get enough fiber in your diet; bran, vegetables, and fruits are rich in fiber.

Congenital spinal cord defects: Inadequate folic acid consumption during pregnancy leads to neural defects in the newborn. Folic acid is usually given as a pill; however, during pregnancy, expectant mothers should eat more legumes, green leafy vegetables, and fruits that are rich in folic acid. This is far more enjoyable than popping pills.

Urinary Tract Infection: Cranberry juice prevents adhesion of bacteria to the walls of the ureter and bladder and thus reduces the incidence of urinary infection. So eat cranberries or drink a glass of cranberry juice daily.

Overall, enough evidence now shows that consuming foods containing more fruits, vegetables, and fiber can reduce the risk of cancer and heart disease. Once again the message comes through loud and clear: eat intelligently, and you will live longer.

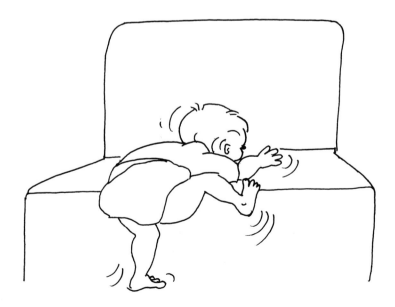

What Will You Be
When You Grow Up?

One day I asked Susan, "What will you be when you grow up?"

She shrugged and said in a cute way, "I don't know".

I had known her since she was eight years old. She had big button eyes with thick eyelashes and her face was pretty and innocent. Susan had two other sisters with different last names. Sometimes all of them used to come to my office with a cold or minor ailment. They would chitchat with me, and leave with smiles, always appreciating what I had done for them. I still remember those visits.

When Susan was in junior high, she had an argument with a classmate that flared into verbal abuse and ended in a fistfight. Susan got a black eye and I treated that.

A couple of years passed by. Susan wasn't doing well at school. One day somebody saw her hiding something behind the bushes before entering school. It turned out to be a beer can, and she was suspended for a few days. Susan was also seen smoking near the school. Her family was already being counseled and child protective services were also involved. Susan's mother told me all this; she seemed to be sincere and very concerned.

I came to know several things about the family by and by. The smiles and the sweet talk from Susan's mother were a facade to hide deep-rooted problems. She was an alcoholic and rarely bothered to check what her children did at school or whether they did their homework. The refrigerator held more beer cans than milk or juice cartons. There was no father in the house, and her boyfriends were more interested in sharing the few dollars and the beer she provided than in committing to the family.

Susan stayed with a foster mother for some time, but one day she ran away with her boyfriend and did not bother to inform anybody. After a couple of days they found her at a near by city.

I checked her for signs of abuse, venereal disease, and drugs. There were none. Susan was moved to a juvenile home with a monitor attached to her so that they could keep track of her whereabouts. About this time she stopped coming to me.

Months later I was called to the hospital nursery to see a newborn baby girl with tremors. The mother had dropped into the birthing center and had had little prenatal care. Tremors in a newborn can be due to low blood sugar, low calcium, low magnesium, infections, etc., and I quickly ruled them out by doing appropriate tests. However, a drug-screening test on the baby's urine showed cocaine metabolites. The mother had taken cocaine, her fetus had been exposed to the drug, and was already addicted in the womb. As soon as it was born, the baby lacked the supply of cocaine, and developed withdrawal symptoms. What a way to start life!

I went to the mother's room to explain what was then going on. Her face seemed very familiar to me—it was Susan.

Soon the baby developed diarrhea, was not sucking well, and slept poorly. I started her on phenobarbital elixir to counteract the effects of the withdrawal symptoms.

What does cocaine do to the unborn child? It can cause congenital malformations like heart defects, skull defects, and kidney-ureter-bladder defects. Cocaine causes high blood pressure in the mother, which leads to the constriction of the blood vessels in the placenta and thus the fetus doesn't get enough oxygen. Possibly that is how some birth defects are produced. Cocaine and amphetamine addiction may cause spontaneous abortion, early placental separation, and fetal distress. Infants who are exposed to cocaine are at very high risk for Sudden Infant Death, the so-called "crib deaths". Long-term disabilities such as attention deficit disorders, concentration difficulties, abnormal play patterns, and apathetic mood disorders have been described in children who have been exposed to cocaine by their mothers.

Please don't take drugs, at least for your children's sake!

The baby did not go home with Susan but was placed in fostercare. The last I saw of the child, she was doing fine, but I can't predict what behavioral problems will crop up in future. She has her mother's big innocent eyes, and I almost asked her one day, "Hello, little Susan! What will *you* be when you grow up?"

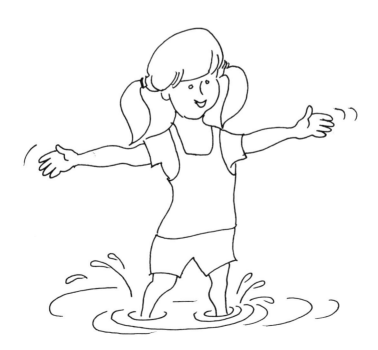

Mom, How Could You
Do This to Me?

ichael is three years old and comes to my office with his grandparents, as his mother's whereabouts are not known. Michael is short for his age and underweight. He is nervous and gets frightened easily. He speaks very few words but communicates by pointing to things. When he was two, Michael had poor motor coordination and walked clumsily, but is better now. Michael's overall development is delayed; he goes to a special school.

Developmental delay can be due to various causes, and after appropriate investigation we ruled out hormonal, chromosomal, and infectious causes in Michael. An MRI scan of the brain showed changes consistent with a migrational abnormality.

What is migrational abnormality, and what is wrong with Michael? Michael's problem could be traced to events that had happened while he was nestling in his mother's womb. During the early stages of brain development, embryonic nerve cells called neuroblasts crawl various distances to form different parts. Some form compact areas called nuclei. Some neuroblasts form loosely woven areas called reticular systems. Yet other neuroblasts migrate to the surface of the primitive brain to form the cerebral cortex, the seat of intelligence. Any chemical or infectious injury can cause abnormal migration of the neuroblasts; the child may suffer various developmental disabilities.

We are beginning to understand the ill effects of drugs like alcohol, cocaine, and others on the developing nervous system. Michael's mother used cocaine during pregnancy, but I'm not sure whether she also used alcohol. Both substances interfere with the normal migration of nerve cells, and this is probably the cause of Michael's problem.

In addition to developmental delays, children exposed to cocaine in the womb can develop urogenital malformations, increased muscle tone, abnormal behaviors, and autistic features. We are not yet sure about the nature of damage caused by multiple drug usage and its long-term effects.

I wish one day Michael could find his mother and ask, "Mom, how could you do this to me?"

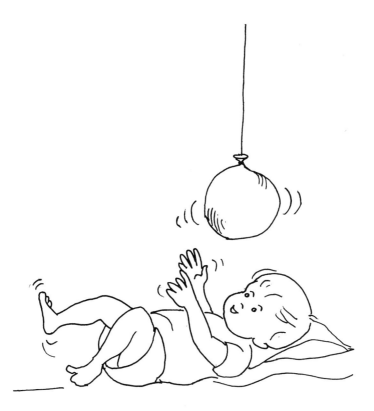

Get Up and Get Involved

*W*hen Mrs. Britts, Chad's foster mother, brought him in for a checkup, he was just five days old and had been born at a hospital in a neighboring town. Mrs. Britts had inherited him from another foster parent the previous day, and did not know much about Chad's mother or his birth history.

I examined Chad, a cute baby, who was well nourished and alert. Now and then he had jittery movements of his extremities that lasted a few seconds. While examining his heart, I found a long "ooosh" sound between the first and the second heart sounds. This condition, called a systolic murmur, could represent a congenital malformation of the heart or its blood vessels. For example, a hole in the heart between the right and left chambers, or a narrowing of the blood vessels like the aorta or pulmonary artery, could cause such a murmur.

There were a few other possibilities. Because this murmur could represent a serious heart condition, I referred Chad to a cardiologist. He found that Chad had a narrowing of his pulmonary artery, the blood vessel that carries impure blood to the lungs for oxygenation. When blood flowed through this narrow opening, the turbulence that was created produced the heart murmur. Chad had a heart condition called pulmonary stenosis. Why did this five-day-old child develop it?

In 1957, a German firm patented and introduced a drug called Thalidomide. It was a sedative and sleep-inducing drug, and many pregnant women took it for sleeplessness. Later, hundreds of babies were born without arms, legs, toes, or fingers and other body parts; they were called "Thalidomide Babies". Consequently,

Thalidomide was withdrawn from the market.

Ever since that incident, when checking a child with congenital malformations, doctors question the mother for possible ingestion of drugs, especially in the first three months of pregnancy during which the cells of the fetus multiply rapidly and differentiate to form various organs. These rapidly replicating cells are vulnerable to any drug or radiation, and such damage could result in malformation of the infant.

Through Mrs. Britt, with some difficulty, I contacted the other foster mother. She did not know much, either. However, the little information she gave me was significant. Chad's teenage mother abused cocaine and alcohol during her entire pregnancy.

Maternal use of cocaine during pregnancy can cause decreased weight, height, and head circumference in the newborn child. Even though rare, brain defects, cystic spaces, kidney abnormalities, limb deformities, and heart lesions can occur due to this drug. I felt Chad's pulmonary stenosis was due to his mother's use of cocaine during pregnancy.

The last time I saw Chad, he was doing well. He did not need any operation. However, he needed to be put on antibiotics every time he visited a dentist or for any minor surgery. His birth mother had counseling and Chad finally went to live with her, where he rightfully belongs.

How bad is drug and alcohol abuse? The statistics are appalling. National studies have shown that 50 percent of students in high school have used a drug at one time or another, 90 percent have taken alcohol and over 35 percent are binge drinkers.

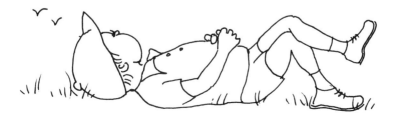

How do these drugs affect all of us? Drugs and alcohol slowly destroy the user economically, psychologically, and socially. Motor vehicular accidents, homicides and suicides are much more frequent among drug users. It is not just family members who suffer—our society pays for the enormous expenses involved in treating the drug abuser's medical, psychological, and rehabilitation programs. Hence it is imperative for you as a parent to recognize early the signs of drug abuse in your teenager and try to prevent it.

What are these early signs? Your son or daughter may become isolated from the family physically and emotionally, spending a lot of time alone in his or her room, or outside the house. Conflicts with you and other family members arise about simple things. School grades may fall; absenteeism and disciplinary problems at school may surface. Your teenager may drop old friends and acquire new ones, who probably use drugs. He or she may lose jobs without reason, have vague complaints, eat poorly and sleep less. Lying, anger, and very selfish behavior may be noted. Stealing in stores and other criminal activities may be brought to your notice. You may find needle marks on him or her; you may find citations for driving under intoxication, needles and syringes or even drugs in your teenager's room.

Teen drug abuse is often associated with parental drug use. Parents shouldn't think they are smart and that their drug use hasn't been noticed by anybody in the family. Unless parents set a good example, lecturing to teenagers about drugs is hypocrisy. The truth of the matter is that you always know the right thing to do. The hard part is doing it.

As a parent, once you suspect or find evidence of drug abuse, make sure you talk to your doctor about your teenager. Get involved in counseling sessions. Your participation proves to your teenager that you care and are serious about his or her welfare. The doctor may refer your teenager and you to a psychologist;

your teenager may also be referred to a drug rehabilitation program. You may be very uncomfortable about these referrals, but make sure you keep the appointments. Don't deny the problem or hope that it will vanish by itself; there is nothing harder than the softness of indifference.

The majority of teenage drug users do not end up as drug abusing adults. As a parent, getting actively involved and supporting your teenager in the difficult and demanding counseling sessions will go a long way towards achieving that goal.

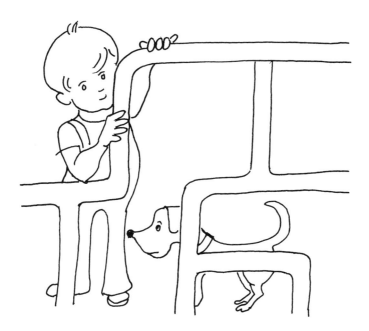

Mystery of the Tylenol Overdose

Many years ago, Stan, then 17 years old, was brought to the emergency room with severe nausea, abdominal cramps, and confusion. Stan told the ER physician that he had developed a severe headache while partying with his friends, and taken one tablet of extra-strength Tylenol. Because the headache did not abate, he then swallowed a few more tablets. Stan experienced severe abdominal cramps and felt he might have taken too much Tylenol. That's why he was brought to the emergency room.

The ER physician passed a tube into Stan's stomach and cleaned it out, removing any residual Tylenol. He promptly drew blood for several laboratory tests including one for an acetaminophen level, a chemical present in Tylenol. The level of the chemical was high in Stan, indicating that he had acetaminophen poisoning. He was started on an antidote called mucomyst, and since there was a distinct possibility that his liver could become severely damaged, he was transferred to a university hospital for further care.

Acetaminophen overdose causes nausea and vomiting for the first one to two days. On the third or fourth day, it damages the liver; sometimes it affects the heart, kidneys, and brain. One in five children die if the liver is damaged severely.

Stan was hooked up to a cardiac monitor and treated with mucomyst and intravenous fluids. His blood acetaminophen levels, kidney functions, and liver parameters were followed closely. The acetaminophen level came down the next day, but liver enzymes were elevated, indicating moderate damage to his liver. Slowly they too came down. Stan was getting better. I felt very happy.

Meanwhile, because ingestion of Tylenol could have been suicidal, a social worker, a psychologist, and a crisis management team were involved in Stan's care. That was very appropriate.

Why did Stan take so many Tylenol pills for a headache? He said his headache was so severe, he swallowed several pills and lost count of how many he had taken.

Meanwhile, his blood when screened for drugs tested positive for tetrahydrocannabinol (THC), a chemical found in marijuana. With this fact in mind we spoke to Stan again. He confessed that he had been smoking a joint at the party.

THC in marijuana is rapidly absorbed by the nasal route and produces its effect in ten minutes. There is elation and euphoria; the person loses critical judgment, develops visual hallucinations, and a distortion of time perception. Short-term memory is also impaired.

That is exactly what had happened to Stan at the party. He took a tablet of Tylenol for a headache after smoking a joint. Because his memory was distorted, he swallowed 15 extra-strength Tylenol tablets without realizing the consequences. Stan was lucky that he sought prompt medical treatment; moreover, his liver was not severely damaged. If he had taken more pills, he could have died.

Teen parties with alcohol and drugs! Tell me, is it worth your life?

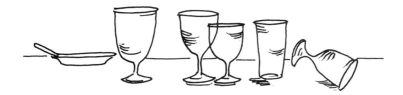

Who Gave You Those Blue Eyes?

One-year-old Melissa was brought to my office for pneumonia. While examining her, I could not help but notice her sky-blue eyes. "Melissa, who gave you those beautiful blue eyes?" I whispered as she crooned and smiled innocently. "Dr. Rao, that's what *I* want to know," said Mrs. Parkinson, Melissa's mother, "I don't have blue eyes; my husband doesn't have blue eyes. How did she get them?"

"Anybody on your husband's side have blue eyes?" I asked.

"A nephew and a niece have blue and hazel eyes," she replied.

"And on your side, do your parents or grandparents have blue eyes?"

"Well, I heard that my great-great-grandfather had blue eyes," she said.

"The blue-eye trait or carrier state is present in both sides of your family. A trait for blue eyes means that the gene is present for blue eyes in a person but he or she will not have blue eyes. I'm sure you and your husband have that trait. When both wife and husband have the trait, 1/4 of their children may be born with blue eyes, and 3/4 will have brown eyes, 2/3 of whom will be carriers for blue eyes. When I say 1/4 of the children may have blue eyes, I mean that during every conception there is a 1-in-4 chance of having a child with blue eyes. This type of transmission of a genetic character or disease is called autosomal recessive inheritance. So you see, Mrs. Parkinson, that while you and your husband can have brown eyes, Melissa can still have blue eyes."

Mrs. Parkinson was very pleased with my explanation.

It is not all so simple. Brown, hazel, or green eyes are inherited as autosomal dominant traits. Blue and gray eyes are inherited as recessive traits. Depending on the genetic makeup of the parents, various shades of eye colors are seen from blue, green, gray, brown, to almost black. There are also eyes with intermediate shades, such as greenish gray, speckled gray, and speckled green. Occasionally, a child with dark-colored eyes is born to parents with light-colored eyes. It is possible that more than one gene controls eye colors.

Once, I examined a five-year-old blue-eyed blonde girl and casually asked her, "Who gave you these beautiful blue eyes, sweetie?"

She looked at me with eyes opened wide in disbelief. "You don't know that, Silly? God gave me my blue eyes!"

True. For Him, who has painted rainbows and given us peacocks, making blue eyes must be a breeze!

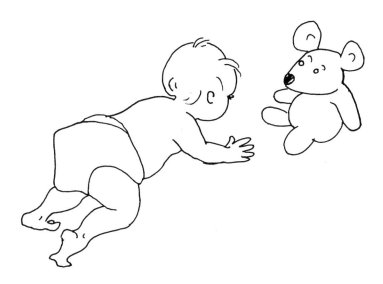

A Minor and Major Blood Problem

$\mathcal{O}$ have known Jonathan since birth. When he was a year old, a routine blood check showed that he was mildly anemic; his hemoglobin stood at 9.9 grams percent, as against a normal range of 11.5 to 15.5 gms percent. Because iron-deficiency anemia is very common at that age, I started Jonathan on iron drops. After a month of treatment, he was still anemic. Jonathan's mother, Mrs. Moreno, swore that she was giving him the iron drops regularly.

I performed several tests on Jonathan to find out why he was anemic. There was no blood loss in the stools. Because children of that age keep everything in their mouths, I tested Jonathan for lead levels; flakes of old house paints contain lead, and eating them could cause lead poisoning and anemia. However, Jonathan's blood did not reveal lead poisoning. His total body iron and serum iron levels were also normal; there was no iron deficiency. So, what was causing the anemia?

Hemoglobin is the iron-containing protein in the blood that carries oxygen to various parts of the body and returns carbon dioxide to the lungs. Adults and children above the age of one year have two kinds of hemoglobin, called A1 and A2. About 96.5 percent of the hemoglobin is of A1 type, and 1.5 to 3.5 percent is of the A2. Hemoglobin A1 has two pairs of polypeptide chains, called alpha and beta chains. Hemoglobin A2 also has two pairs of chains, called alpha and delta. If a genetic defect affects the beta chain synthesis, hemoglobin A1 cannot be produced in normal amounts and the level of hemoglobin A2 is increased in the blood. Thus, an elevated hemoglobin A2 indicates defective hemoglobin A1 synthesis.

I ordered tests on Jonathan to measure the relative levels of hemoglobin A1 and A2; they showed that his hemoglobin A2 was elevated. He had a genetic defect in producing hemoglobin A1, a defect that is called "Thalassemia Minor or Trait."

Children affected with thalassemia minor are mildly anemic for life but no other problems are noticed. This disease is often mistaken for iron-deficiency anemia. Sometimes iron is given for prolonged periods unnecessarily; the anemia will not improve as the defect is not due to iron deficiency.

When both parents have thalassemia traits, each pregnancy carries a 25 percent risk of a child being born with a severe blood defect called "Thalassemia Major". This is a terrible disease; affected children have severe anemia requiring repeated lifelong blood transfusions, and most of them die before they are 20.

I stopped Jonathan's iron therapy and assured his mother that the mild anemia would not harm him. I also asked her to get her own and her husband's blood checked for thalassemia. I explained to her at length the genetic implications of thalassemia minor, and also advised her that when Jonathan planned to get married, he should make sure his fiancee didn't have thalassemia minor; otherwise some of their children may inherit the severe disease of thalassemia major.

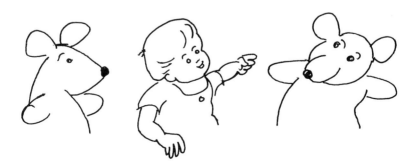

Christmas Disease

*B*randon's mother brought him to my office when he was just three-and-a-half months old. Except for an upper respiratory tract infection, Brandon was well. He had had a tongue-tie at birth and it was snipped off without any bleeding; other than that, he had an uneventful newborn period.

Brandon's family history was very interesting. Brandon's elder brother bruised easily for minor injuries. Brandon's maternal uncle had a bleeding problem, but Brandon's mother was normal, and so also was his sister. There was no history of a bleeding tendency on Brandon's paternal side; it seemed that the bleeding problem was confined to his maternal side and affected only the male members.

As the weeks went by, Brandon too began to show a tendency to bruise easily. At one time, he had vomited a small quantity of blood, but recovered completely.

Why did Brandon bruise and bleed so easily? When a normal child has a cut or injury, he or she stops bleeding in a few minutes; this is because of the property of blood to clot, which is a protective mechanism. Clotting is a very complex process; in simple words, a clot consists of interwoven threads of a substance called fibrin, with platelets, red cells, and white cells entangled in that mesh. Fibrin is derived from another glycoprotein called fibrinogen. For fibrinogen to be converted to fibrin, another substance called thrombin is necessary; this, in turn, is derived from prothrombin. In order for prothrombin to get converted to thrombin, many substances called "factors" are needed. These include factors VIII, IX, X, XI, XII, and a few others. If any one factor is missing, prothrombin cannot form thrombin. In the absence of thrombin, fibrinogen cannot be converted to fibrin, a decent clot cannot form, and the person bleeds.

Brandon had factor IX deficiency, which is called hemophilia B. This ailment is also known as Christmas disease, coined after a five-year-old boy named Christmas who was among the first patients in whom this condition was diagnosed. Christmas disease is inherited as a sex-linked recessive disorder; females carry and transmit the disease but usually don't have problems. Affected male children may have no problems, or may develop various degrees of a bleeding tendency, depending on the level of factor IX in the blood. Severely affected children, when they have a minor injury, may bleed into the joints, muscles, and internal organs, occasionally threatening their lives. Doctors used to give fresh frozen plasma to treat severe bleeding. Nowadays, concentrated factor IX is available to alleviate the complications of the disease.

Every Christmas, I am reminded of the Christmas disease and I think of Brandon. The last time I saw him, he was doing well without major bleeding problems, thanks to the treatments he received with purified factor IX.

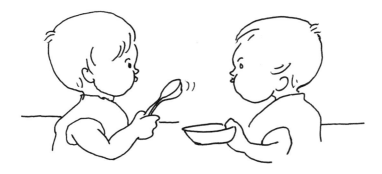

The Human Genome Project—
Useful for Children?

"I discovered a new gene that is responsible for discovering new genes," said a geneticist humorously. The complete set of chromosomes is called the "genome" and its secrets are being revealed at an astonishing pace. The sequence of three billion pairs of nucleotides that form about 100,000 genes has been unveiled by the human genome project (HGP). These genes have the codes that make a human being perfect and imperfect. It is amazing that only four nucleotides—thymine (T), cytosine (C), adenine (A) and guanine (G)—are arranged in varying orders to form this string of life. If we type side by side the letters forming the above four nucleotides in the entire genome, the line will be 3,000 miles long!

How does this genetic map help us to diagnose and treat diseases? Once the sequence of the nucleotides in the genes is known, abnormal sequences can be readily identified by sensitive tests that are being developed. Patterns of disease inheritance will be clarified. Diseases such as diabetes, obesity, and asthma can be diagnosed long before they manifest themselves, and prompt preventive measures can be undertaken.

Here are a couple of pediatric scenarios:

A one-year-old child has a fever and develops seizures. The possibility of a brain infection is ruled out by appropriate tests. Seizures that occur as a result of fever are called "febrile seizures". Researchers have found that three chromosomes harbor genes that cause febrile seizures. By screening other siblings for this gene, their doctor can predict which child will develop seizures and which child will have severe problems that require medication. Parents using this information can avoid emergency room visits.

A two-year-old child develops meningococcal meningitis and gets intravenous antibiotics. Parents ask the doctor whether their child will live and what they should do about the siblings who are exposed to the infection. The doctor orders a genetic analysis of the sick child. The analysis tells him that the child is prone to intravascular coagulation called DIC that could cause death. He promptly starts the child on heparin. Genetic tests on the meningococcus germ show that it has a gene that imparts resistance to the antibiotic being used. The doctor immediately chooses another antibiotic. Meanwhile, the siblings' genetic analysis comes back. One sibling has a gene that favors a carrier state; he is followed with repeated cultures and appropriate antibiotics. Other siblings have normal gene patterns and are given prophylactic antibiotics.

There are other benefits to the HGP. Gene therapy, the method of introducing normal genes into the body of a person who has deficiency of a particular gene, was successful in a disease called adenosine diaminase deficiency. Gene therapy to gonodal tissue, called "germ line gene therapy", is also being done experimentally.

The HGP will dramatically change the way we practice medicine. Molecular diagnostic tests will be available to diagnose genetic disorders. Interesting therapies like gene replacement and cloning of tissues to replace genetically defective organs will become common. Certain genetic disorders that we know now will become extinct.

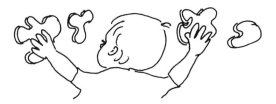

When Deafness Is Inherited

Mina and Dina were twins. I have known them well from their birth until they stopped coming to me at about the age of fifteen. They were always charming, smiling, and beautiful; just from looking at them, you would never guess what their problem was. But if you asked them a question, you would notice that they would carefully watch your lips and answer you in grunts, smiles, and sign language. They could not talk, and they could not hear. They were deaf from birth.

Diseases such as Alport syndrome that affect the kidneys and other organs are also associated with deafness. Some ear malformations can also cause deafness. We eliminated those causes in Mina and Dina by taking a careful medical history and also referring them to several experts.

Because deafness can be inherited, I also took a careful family history. Mina and Dina's parents had normal hearing. The twins maternal aunt had a son who was born deaf. Moreover, their elder sister Susan and a younger sister Monica had congenital deafness. Several years later, when Susan had children, a girl and two boys were deaf. One other boy was normal. What a heartbreaking family history! It appeared as though God were playing a game of dice, affecting some and sparing others.

Because boys as well as girls in the family were affected, the hearing loss seemed to be inherited in an autosomal recessive manner. What does that mean? A disease or a message is said to be autosomal when it is located on a chromosome other than a sex chromosome. The term 'recessive' refers to the fact that we need two abnormal messages to actually get the disease. In Mina and Dina's family, both mom and dad were carrying a normal and a hearing-loss gene, so they were carriers of the disease. However, because they each had one normal gene, their hearing was normal. In Mina, Dina, and other family members who were deaf, mom and dad each gave them a hearing-loss gene. Thus these children inherited two hearing-loss genes, making them deaf.

Normal children in the family inherited one hearing-loss gene and a normal gene or two normal genes from their parents. As long as they had one normal gene, their hearing was unaffected.

Recent research has shown that mutations are common in the connexin 26 and 30 genes, which are responsible for deafness. It is estimated that 2.8 percent of the population carry this mutation gene for deafness, and 1 in 1,000 children are affected with genetic deafness. Nowadays doctors do cochlear transplants to improve hearing for such deaf children.

Several years passed before Dina and Mina joined a school for the deaf near San Francisco and did well. A couple of years later I learned that Dina had become pregnant. I prayed to God that her child should not inherit deafness, but came to know later that the child too, alas, had defective hearing.

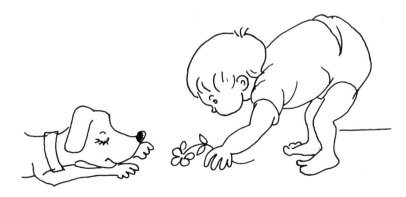

Rare Rings in the Eyes

ohen, 11 years old, was admitted to a hospital with complaints of slurring speech and a tremor of his fingers, which had developed gradually over many months. He also had a weakness in his arms and legs. He denied taking drugs. There was no history of similar illness in the family.

Routine laboratory tests showed a mild anemia and a minimal elevation of his liver enzymes. A neurologist was consulted. Many diseases could cause these symptoms and signs. In those days, CAT scans were experimental and unavailable. A test called a myelogram was performed on Cohen to detect whether a tumor existed in the upper part of the spinal cord or at the brain stem. No tumor was found. We were baffled.

A saying goes that when everything else fails, one reads the instruction manual. I opened a textbook and read. Three salient features were affecting Cohen: his tremor, the slightly elevated liver enzymes indicating that the liver was involved, and anemia. The presence of these three together point to a condition called "Wilson disease". In this disease, abnormal amounts of copper accumulate in various organs, including the eyes, and the copper accumulation can be seen as beautiful red rings around the corneas, called the "Kayser-Fleischer rings (KF rings)." If Cohen had the rings, their presence would confirm that he had Wilson disease.

I picked up a flashlight and shone it directly into Cohen's eyes, but did not see any rings. However, I had his blood tested for a protein called ceruloplasmin; Cohen's ceruloplasmin level was low, a sign that he had Wilson disease.

This disease is very rare, occurring in 1 in 500,000 births.

The patient has a genetic defect in excreting copper. Normally, the liver handles the copper and excretes it in the bile. In Wilson disease, abnormal amounts of copper accumulate in the liver, brain, and other organs. Copper is detrimental to cells and free copper in the blood causes a rupture of red cells; that was why Cohen had tremors, weakness, elevated liver enzymes, and anemia.

By the time the nervous system is involved, children with Wilson disease develop KF rings. How come we didn't see them? We flashed the light again in Cohen's eyes, this time at an angle from the side. There they were, two beautiful shining copper rings, one in each eye! We missed them the first time because I had shined the light directly from the front. It's never too late to learn!

We treated Cohen with a drug that excreted copper, and he gradually improved. By the time he left the hospital, his tremor was almost gone.

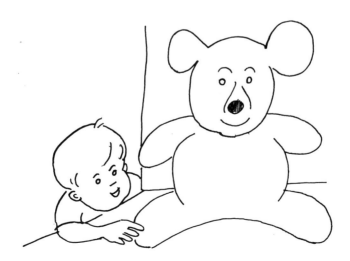

Eat a Potato and Get Immunized!

*I*van was two months old when he was brought to my office for a routine checkup and immunizations. Because he was healthy, I immunized him by giving him three injections. These three shots contained materials to protect him against six diseases, namely, diphtheria, whooping cough, tetanus, poliomyelitis, hemophilus influenzae b, and hepatitis B infections. At the age of four months I gave him the same shots again.

These injections were painful. As Ivan cried, his mother asked me, "Dr. Rao, my baby has become a pincushion. Is there any way you can give him fewer shots? Why can't you give these vaccines by mouth?"

"Except for oral polio, all the other immunizations have to be given by injection," I replied. "In this country, polio vaccine too is given as an injection. Given orally, proteins in most vaccines will be digested and will not give the needed immunity. However, by choosing combinations of the immunizations, we can reduce the number of injections, and that is why I've given Ivan only three."

Even though current vaccines such as DTaP or MMR cannot be given orally, other newer vaccines are being developed that can be given by mouth or through the nose. Particular progress is being made with vaccines that would prevent diarrhea, which is welcome news; worldwide, diarrhea caused by bacteria is a major cause of death in infants. It is estimated that three million deaths occur each year due to bacterial diarrhea, salmonella bacteria being among the causes. Scientists are developing an oral vaccine for this disease; genetically engineered, it will also provide protection against several other diseases caused by germs like E. coli and shigella. An intranasal vaccine that will guard against influenza, the cause of severe respiratory infections and pneumonias in children, has already been developed and is recommended for certain age groups. These new vaccines will be a boon to children.

Medical companies are experimenting with vaccines that are encapsulated in shells to protect against acid in the stomach. Some of the vaccines now given by injection could then be given orally.

Yet another elegant approach is being tried. Plants are genetically altered to synthesize various vaccines. Potato, corn, tomato, alfalfa, lettuce, and spinach can be altered genetically to produce bacterial antigens; when such a vegetable is consumed, it will evoke a response in the body to protect against a disease.

Recently, scientists at the Boyce Thompson Institute for Plant Research have developed a super potato, which has genes incorporated from diarrhea-causing E. coli bacteria. These potatoes are called transgenic potatoes. Under the supervision of Carol O. Tacket, MD, at the University of Maryland School of Medicine, a preliminary six-month study was conducted on 14 healthy adults. Volunteers who ate these potatoes were protected against E. coli infection as evidenced by the development of an antibody against the bacteria both in blood and stools. A few volunteers complained of nausea on eating the altered potatoes; no other side effects were noticed. But the potatoes were raw; cooking them will probably destroy their antigenic property.

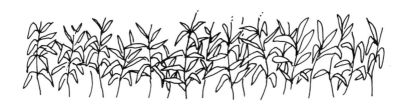

Transgenic plants that could offer protection against other infections such as hepatitis B and rabies are also being developed. These genetically altered vegetables can be grown easily and are cheap, and can be readily shipped to other parts of the country. It is to be hoped that they will be available soon to protect against various diseases. When that happens, you'll be able to sit on a couch with your child, eat potatoes, and get immunized!

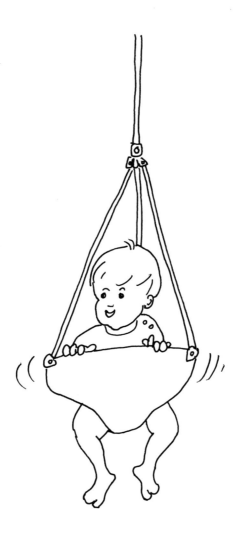

The Smell of Diseases

Mrs. Roberts brought five-year-old Ted to my office with a high fever and a sore throat. During examination, I found that he had tonsillitis with pus; in addition, he had a fine rash all over his body. Because tonsillitis with a rash could be due to a streptococcal infection, I sent a throat swab to the lab for a culture. While I was doing that, Mrs. Robert's commented that Ted's breath was smelling odd.

"When a child has pus in his throat, the breath sometimes smells bad," I said.

"I know that, but this is different," Mrs. Roberts insisted. "Ted has a peculiar odor to his breath."

I did not notice that peculiar odor. I know that children with diabetes mellitus who have a complication of ketoacidosis smell sweet from the acetone. Children with kidney failure also have a peculiar smell. Children with inborn errors of amino acid metabolism secrete abnormal substances in their urine or sweat; they smell like maple syrup, cabbage, or rotting fish. Some have the smell of a mouse or tomcat's urine. But a sore throat with a peculiar smell?

I had read an article that described a distinct breath odor in children with streptococcal infections. The investigators found that this odor was present in 4 to 5 percent of children who had the infection. The positive predictive value of this suspicious smell was 72.7 percent; in other words, if a child with a sore throat has a breath with a peculiar smell, that child very likely is suffering from streptococcal sore throat.

Scientists, using techniques such as gas chromatography, are studying the odors that various diseases emit. By measuring the odors in exhaled air, special instruments can detect the type of bacteria infecting a person. The day is not far off when a child will just need to breathe into the tube of a machine, and in a few seconds the machine will announce, "Ted, your breath analysis shows that you have a streptococcus group A infection. The preferred antibiotic to use is…."

Ted's throat culture came back positive for streptococcus group A. Mrs. Roberts was right about the peculiar odor. As always, mothers know best.

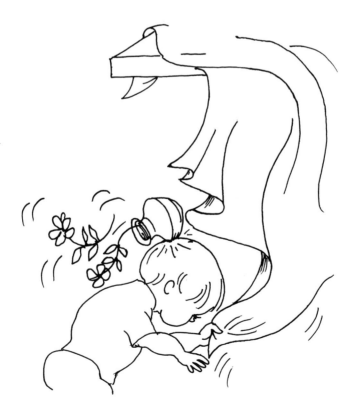

Cold Facts

"Nathan gets colds every 15 days. Can't you do something about it, Dr. Rao?" Mrs. Perkins said to me. "Nathan has neither allergies nor immune problems," I told her. "I've checked him for both. But he does go to a daycare center; it's likely that he gets infections there."

"So many times?"

"Rhinoviruses are one out of more than 200 different kinds that can cause common colds," I pointed out. "Since there are 101 serologically different rhinoviruses, and one does not develop lasting immunity to any of them, theoretically one can get infected endlessly."

She made a face. "Perhaps you can give him an antibiotic?"

"Drugs that kill the viruses are called antiviral agents. They don't work well for common colds."

"Why not?" Mrs. Perkins asked.

Recently I read about a study on the common cold by Dr. Turner and others. Dr. Turner selected 18 healthy volunteers. After making sure that they didn't have transient immunity to the rhinovirus, each of them was infected with rhinovirus type 23 by squirting it into their noses. Then they were kept in isolation. Once they got infected, the participants kept a strict log of their signs and symptoms. They noted how many times they sneezed, coughed, blew their noses, had chills and headaches, and so on; they even weighed the Kleenexes to measure the amount of mucous secreted. The mucous was then analyzed for chemicals, enzymes, and substances such as interleukins (ILs) and cytokinins that are produced when there is inflammation. After four days of this exhausting human experiment, the study was completed.

What did Dr. Turner find out after this experiment? It seems the rhinovirus infects surprisingly very few cells in the nasal mucous membrane. The infected cells produce substances such as interleukin-8 (IL-8) and cytokinins. These substances attract white cells, which produce an inflammatory response characterized by nasal discharge, sneezing, and other symptoms of a cold. So it is not the virus that causes the symptoms, but the body's reaction to IL-8. If IL-8 is not produced, there are no symptoms of a cold, even though the person has been infected with the rhinovirus. By the time one has a runny nose, the inflammatory reaction has already started, and it is too late to take an antiviral agent. One has to suffer patiently.

"Mrs. Perkins," I said, "medical companies are trying to develop drugs that inhibit IL-8 production. The day is not far off when, after an overnight party where you were exposed to someone with a cold, you'll take a pill next morning that inhibits IL-8 production, thus preventing the inflammatory response and the cold symptoms. A morning-after-pill for a cold!"

Mrs. Perkins laughed heartily.

I prescribed Nathan a decongestant and sent him home.

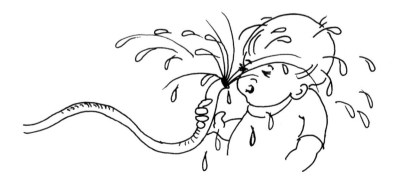

New Skin for Old

When summer is around the corner, and families head for the beach or the park and suntans, you probably know that the sun's ultraviolet rays are harmful and cause mutations in the DNA of skin cells; this leads to cancers such as melanoma, and basal and squamous cell carcinomas. Still, you want the children to have their share of fun; what can you do to protect them? Normally, enzymes called endonucleases, that are present in cells, initiate the repair process, handling any damage to the DNA; other enzymes then take over and complete the repair. This goes on constantly; but sometimes, the sun's rays cause damage too fast for the natural healing process to catch up. Can the damage caused by UV rays be reversed promptly? Can old skin be exchanged for new?

Researchers are working on a skin lotion that has the magic effect of rejuvenating damaged skin. The lotion has liposomes, microscopic oil bubbles full of a viral enzyme that can repair damaged DNA. This enzyme is called T4 endonuclease V. When the lotion is applied to the skin, the liposomes enter the skin cells. There, the enzyme endonuclease V is released from the vesicles and enters the nucleus, combines with the damaged DNA strands and starts the repair process.

Other enzymes also enhance repair. Cyanobacteria produce an enzyme called photolyase that reduces DNA damage by 40 percent. Another bacterium called micrococcus luteus harbors a protein akin to endonuclease V. These enzymes and proteins are patented and made available, for a price, to manufacturers of skin lotions and cremes. Do these products help?

A medical condition called *xeroderma pigmentosa* is an inherited disease where children who are affected become very sensitive to sunlight. They lack an enzyme to repair damage to skin cells caused by ultra-violet light. These children cannot come out into sunlight and venture out only at night; they are called "children of the moon". In such children, scientists have tried the DNA-repair enzyme-containing lotion. Children who received treatment for a year had decreased incidence of basal cell carcinoma and actinic keratosis, a precancerous lesion, proving that the lotion is beneficial. Now, clinical trials are underway in people who have a family history of skin cancer. A lotion or cream will be available soon that will enhance the repair process of the damaged skin and thus perhaps decrease the incidence of skin cancers.

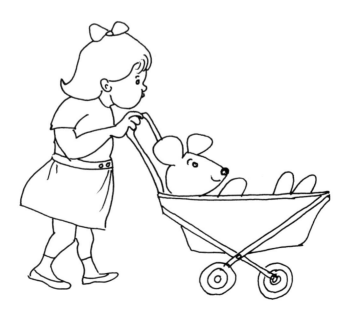

Scorpion and Cancer

*N*o, I'm not talking about astrology signs. Oscar, ten years old, attended Camp Scicon; while standing and chatting with friends near a pile of rocks and dried leaves, Oscar felt a sting in his foot. As he jerked his foot away thinking it was a bee, he noticed a strange crawling creature that he and his friends had never seen before. One of his friends said it was a spider; another said it was a big red ant or a scorpion. While they were discussing the various possibilities, the creature scuttled under a pile of dried leaves and disappeared.

Oscar's foot hurt and itched for a few hours. The next day he came to see me along with his mother. He did not have any complications from the sting. By that time he knew the creature that stung him was a scorpion.

"Why didn't you kill it?" I asked.

"We didn't know what it was, and it was so cute!" replied Oscar.

More than 1,000 species of scorpion are found worldwide. In California, a scorpion called *centruroides elixicada* can cause problems. Most stings cause local reactions such as mild burning or severe pain. Within a few hours other symptoms like agitation, salivation, blurred vision, high blood pressure, rapid breathing, and fast heart rate may develop. Small children may suffer from respiratory failure, convulsions, and coma. In other parts of the globe, scorpion poison can affect the muscles, heart, and the nervous system, causing death.

The darkest cloud has a silver lining: the deadly poison has an interesting beneficial effect. Recently it was found that the venom of the giant Israeli scorpion has the capacity to seek and cripple the cells of a brain cancer called glioma. So far there has been no effective treatment for this cancer, but scorpion venom has a neurotoxin called chlorotoxin, which specifically attacks 98 percent of the glioma cells, immobilizes them, and thus prevents their spread. While chlorotoxin itself does not kill the cancer cells, scientists are able to kill the cancer cells effectively by attaching a cell-killing-protein to the chlorotoxin.

How did the scientists get the idea to check the scorpion venom? Scorpion venom paralyzes and kills insects such as crickets and cockroaches. The ability of the venom to enter the nervous system attracted the attention of scientists who thought they might use it to treat brain cancer.

I told Oscar that he should have sought medical help immediately after the sting. But it was good that Oscar was not a scorpion-killer. We need scorpions to cure cancer!

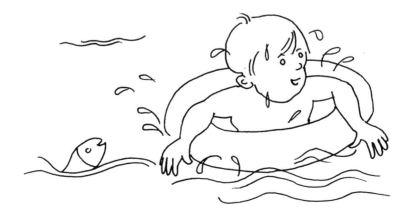

Behind Every Man's Success

*W*hen Brenda developed pain in her hips, I requested several X rays. She had recovered from a cancer of her lymph nodes, and her hip pain could be due to a recurrence of the cancer. Naturally her mother was very worried about it and the ill effects of radiation. I spoke to a radiologist who assured me that the radiation from each X ray was less than a rad and that this small amount would not cause any damage.

I conveyed this message to Brenda's mother, who now felt comfortable. Moreover the X rays showed no evidence of cancer but did reveal a degeneration of Brenda's hipbones. No wonder doctors find X rays a valuable tool in diagnosing diseases.

An interesting story lies behind the discovery of X rays. Early in 1885, William Conrad Roentgen was conducting experiments with a Crookes tube. These tubes, which were named after their inventor, the English physicist Sir William Crookes, were vacuum glass cylinders containing electrodes through which an electric current could be passed. Various rays, emitted under different experimental conditions, were being studied during that time. One of the rays emitted from the Crookes tube made chemically coated plates glow, a process we now call fluorescence. It was also known that these particular rays, that we now call cathode rays, were weak and had their effect only up to a few inches from the tube.

Roentgen was curious whether the cathode rays could pass through opaque objects. One day, he covered the Crookes tube with an opaque cardboard and closed all the curtains in the laboratory to avoid any effect from the outside light. When he passed an electric current through the tube, he noticed a bright greenish-yellow colored flame flickering about a yard from the Crookes tube. He thought he was hallucinating, but on opening the curtains he noticed another chemically coated cardboard lying at the very spot where he noted the flickering flame of color. He repeated the experiment several times and observed the same phenomenon. The cardboard fluoresced even when it was moved farther out by several yards. Roentgen surmised that this effect was not due to the cathode rays, but to some other mysterious rays. He named them X rays.

Roentgen began experimenting with the X rays. On November 8, 1895, he placed a deck of cards and a two-inch-thick book between the chemically coated cardboard and the tube. He observed the fluorescence again. It was now clear that the X rays could pass through opaque objects. He tested various materials and found that X rays did not pass through lead but passed easily through wood. Nowadays, technicians and radiologists wear aprons with lead to protect themselves against radiation.

In December, Roentgen held a small lead pipe between a photographic plate and the Crookes tube. When he developed the film he saw not only the shadow of the lead pipe but also the bones of his fingertips holding the pipe. The X rays could pass through flesh but not through the bones. This finding stunned him.

One day he invited his wife, Bertha, to his laboratory, and asked her to place her left hand on a photographic plate lying in a lightproof wooden cassette. She was apprehensive when the Crookes tube flashed and crackled as the current passed through the electrodes. After six minutes of exposure, he developed the film. When he showed her the X ray picture revealing her finger bones, Bertha cried, "Oh my God, I'm seeing my bones. I feel I'm looking at my own death."

Roentgen wrote a paper about the X rays and his experiments and sent it to a physical-medical society. The editor was about to reject the manuscript, but when he saw the X ray picture of the finger bones, he accepted the paper and published it in a medical journal. Soon, newspapers picked up the news and spread it all over Europe. People could not believe that their bones could be seen when they were still alive. They even worried that the most intimately hidden parts could be exposed. Many fainted when they saw their skull bones revealed in detail. Soon, broken bones, bullets, and other objects were being detected with X rays, aiding in diagnosis and treatment.

Roentgen received the Nobel Prize for discovering X rays and he was the first one to receive the prize in physics—all this because his wife let him X ray her hand. One more proof, if proof is needed, that a woman's helping hand lies behind every man's success!

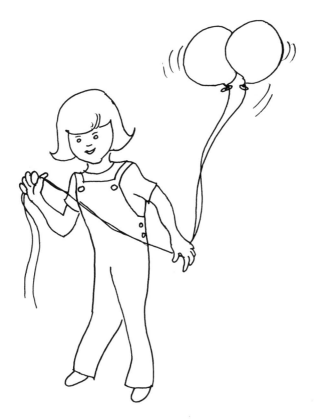

The Incredible Story of Insulin

*K*en, an eight-year-old boy, had diabetes that was poorly controlled, so the doctors at a nearby diabetic clinic gave him a pump that delivered exact amounts of insulin at specific times. Ken excitedly showed me the pump—it meant that he no longer needed to be poked with needles in order to get his correct dose.

Diabetes mellitus is an age-old disease and insulin still remains the main treatment of choice for many diabetic patients. Who discovered insulin and how?

In 1899 Oscar Minkowski and Joseph von Mering were studying the role of the pancreas in digestion (the pancreas is an organ in the abdomen that lies cuddled in the arms of the duodenum, the first part of the small intestine). The two scientists removed the pancreas of a dog. Later, the laboratory technician reported that flies gathered in numbers around the animal's cage, so the scientists tested the dog's urine for sugar by collecting it in a saucer and placing it on a windowsill. If flies gathered around the saucer, it meant that sugar was present in the urine. This was further confirmed by tasting the urine for sweetness. This was how diabetes was diagnosed in those days. Minkowski and von Mering then proved that when the pancreas was removed, the dog developed diabetes and died.

Minkowski and von Mering conducted another experiment. Having tied the pancreatic duct of a dog, they observed that the dog became emaciated but did not develop diabetes. They concluded that the non-glandular part of the pancreas produced a substance that prevented diabetes; the glandular part produced a digestive enzyme.

In 1909, Opie and MacCallum of Johns Hopkins University conducted many experiments on dogs, and concluded that the tail portion of the pancreas produced a substance that prevented the development of diabetes mellitus. They named it "insulin".

About 1920, a young graduate named Frederick G. Banting from the University of Toronto got a job offer in the physiology department of the University of Western Ontario, also in Canada. Preparing for his lectures on diabetes, Banting read that insulin could not be isolated because an enzyme in the pancreas—now we know it as trypsin—digested the insulin during extraction. Banting also studied the Minkowski and von Mering experiment of tying the pancreatic ducts of dogs, who consequently did not develop diabetes. Banting surmised that the enzyme-producing glandular portion withered away, leaving behind the insulin-producing parts. He thought over these experiments and could not sleep well. One day at 2 A.M., he wrote in his notebook, "Ligate the pancreatic ducts of dogs. Wait 6 to 8 weeks for degeneration of glandular cells. Then remove the remaining pancreas and extract insulin."

With these ideas in mind, Banting canceled his trip to his new post. Instead, he approached Dr. Maclead, Professor of Physiology at the University of Toronto, to use his facility to conduct experiments. Dr. Maclead agreed and offered to help. Two medical students were available at that time, and Dr. Maclead said that only one of them could assist Dr. Banting. The students flipped a coin; Charles H. Best was thus chosen by chance to be Dr. Banting's assistant.

By summer's end in 1921, Banting and Best had a pancreatic extract (insulin) that lowered blood sugar. Later, they created diabetic dogs and treated them with insulin and kept them alive. By January 1922, they had a preparation pure enough to use on humans. Banting and Best selected a 14 year-old boy who weighed only 65 pounds because of dietary restrictions. With insulin injections, the boy gained weight and his blood and urine sugar showed improvement. After two weeks, when the treatment was stopped, he worsened within a short time. When he was given insulin again, he improved. Thus, Banting and Best proved the efficacy of insulin in treating patients with diabetes mellitus.

Banting and Maclead were awarded the Nobel Prize in physiology; Banting shared his prize with Best.

Later the Eli Lilly Company took over the task of manufacturing insulin. It is interesting to note that pancreases from 6,000 cattle or 24,000 hogs were required to produce just an ounce of insulin. Nowadays, human insulin is manufactured by bacteria that have been genetically altered.

There is a sequel to the Nobel Prize story. In 1923, just a year after Banting and Best had improved their pancreatic extract, Dr. George Minot, a 36-year-old Boston physician who had diabetes mellitus found himself on the verge of a diabetic coma. He was one of the first few patients who received insulin. He lived to do pioneering work on pernicious anemia and saved many lives with his liver extract injections. Dr. Minot himself received the Nobel Prize in 1934. Without insulin, he probably would not have survived to either earn the prize or to receive it.

Banting and Best. Two scientists best remembered in the incredible story of insulin.

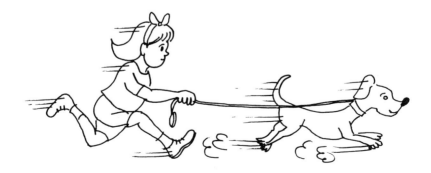

Viva B-Sensor! Viva E-Nose!

Mrs. Williams was visibly worried about her ten-day-old premature infant, Gary. "We had a party last night, Dr. Rao. Everyone was kissing Gary," she said. "Is there a way to know whether Gary was exposed to the flu or any other infection?"

I could understand Mrs. Williams' concern.

"Because newborns have low immunity, they are sitting ducks for infections," I replied. "It is best to avoid parties. There's nothing wrong in asking friends and relatives who have colds and coughs to keep away from Gary. However, because you are nursing the baby, you are giving him an immunity that will probably prevent any serious infection."

Mrs. Williams' question about whether there are ways to detect exposure to infections is very timely. Devices such as biosensors (b-sensors) and electronic noses (e-noses) are even now being developed to detect infections, but they are still at an experimental stage.

The biosensor is a hand-held device. The heart of the device is a bioagent chip, a 2.5 cm square made of plastic. The chip has a minute winding groove to facilitate the flow of air and microfluids. On this groove, there are several tiny 1 to 2 mm squares, each square harboring 10,000 B cells. These B cells are mouse lymphocytes that are sensitized to different pathogens, such as influenza, and fungi. When a virus particle floating in the air comes into contact with the B cells in the sensor, it induces an antigen-antibody reaction that can easily be detected by bioluminescence. The culprit is identified based on the group of B cells that shows luminescence. Because the antigen-antibody reactions are very specific, the b-sensor is highly sensitive. Just ten viral particles are enough to induce a reaction. In the future, doctors may carry this device to detect virus and other infections.

The electronic devices called e-noses are being developed to detect subtle odors of bacteria. For example, one experimental e-nose detected six of the seven bacteria causing urinary tract infections. As the technology advances, portable e-noses will be available to detect most of the infectious and metabolic diseases.

The day is not far off when a concerned mother like Mrs. Williams will carry a small e-nose (probably not as cute as a human nose) or b-sensor in her purse. After a party at her home is over, she will access the Internet using the same device and request an analysis of the sampled air. Back will come the reply about all the viruses and bacteria that members of the family were exposed to, and the precautions and medications they should take.

Viva b-sensor! Viva e-nose!

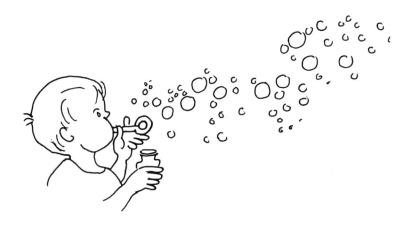

A Clever Mouse

"$\mathcal{D}$r. Rao, we have an unwelcome visitor. Have a look!" my secretary said, excitedly. I opened a door cautiously and peeked inside the room and saw a cute little mouse dashing around. My secretary promptly jumped onto a table screaming, "Catch it, catch it!" I grabbed an empty box in hopes of somehow luring the mouse into it. With astonishing agility, the little mouse slid behind the refrigerator and disappeared.

We consider mice to be vermin. However, mice have contributed enormously to our understanding of human diseases, including infections, cancers, and genetic disorders. Mice are well suited for medical experiments because they are easily available and most of their genes have similar human gene counterparts. Mice can be rapidly reproduced in specialized laboratories. One pair of mice can produce 250 descendants in a year. About 25 million mice are reproduced a year for scientific purposes. Because mice can be bred fast, they can be reproduced easily with special characteristics. By careful manipulation, they have been reproduced with tumor susceptibilities, albinism, Alzheimer's disease, and other ailments. Some mice called "knockout" strains are generated by deleting one or two genes from their chromosomes. Such mice are suitable for studying diseases resulting from gene deletions and are used to test gene therapy. Thus more than 2,500 specialized strains of mice are available currently for scientific experiments.

Some strains of mice are very hard to produce; they require a germ-free atmosphere, special diets, and techniques like cloning. Some of these strains have been patented and are expensive to buy. For example, a hairless flesh-tone mouse with impaired immunity will cost about $75. In contrast, some very rare breeds of genetically altered mice cost $30,000 a pair!

What is the advantage of having so many varieties of mice? If one wants to test a new drug for diabetes, it is unethical to do so on a human being. However, one can custom-order diabetic mice and test the new drug on them. Mice with specific cancers can be ordered to study the effects of anti-cancer drugs. There is practically no limit to the diversity of experiments that can be carried out on the mice.

Manipulating the mice to study diseases is one thing, but genetically altering mice to make them more intelligent is another. Recently, mice were genetically engineered to make more of a protein subunit called the N-methyl-D-aspartate (NMDA) receptor. This NMDA receptor strengthens the connection between neurons, which, simplistically put, is the fundamental mechanism of learning and memory. These mice were able to recognize objects better than normal mice. Their memory also was longer lasting, in that they could remember the location of a platform in a murky water tank. Since these mice were smarter, they were called Doogie mice, named after the genius boy on a once-popular television program, *Doogie Howser, M.D.*

Even though it will take some time, drugs are being developed that act on NMDA receptors to enhance memory and intelligence. Successful experiments with mice now raise the question of whether we could produce superintelligent children by genetic manipulation. This kind of research will change our future in interesting and unpredictable ways. I never caught the mouse in my office. Now I know why. It was a Doogie mouse!

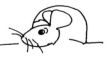

New Treatments for Hemophilia

eter's knee swelled with blood soon after he bumped into a chair. This was not unusual as Peter had a bleeding disorder known as hemophilia. In this disease, a protein called factor VIII is diminished or absent in the blood. Factor VIII and a few other factors are essential for blood clotting, which prevents excessive bleeding after a cut or injury. In patients with hemophilia, even a minor trauma will cause severe bleeding. That was what had happened to Peter.

Hemophilia is a very interesting disease that can be diagnosed by simple blood tests; prenatally, it can even be diagnosed by DNA analysis. Women carry the disease and have no bleeding problems; however, each male child born to a mother with the hemophilia gene has a 50 percent chance of inheriting the disease.

I admitted Peter to a hospital in the morning, applied a pressure bandage to his knee to prevent further bleeding, and ordered a blood product called "cryoprecipitate" that is prepared in blood banks from plasma and is rich in factor VIII. When infused into the blood stream, cryoprecipitate corrects the factor VIII deficiency and stops the bleeding. In those days, the cryoprecipitate had to be transported from a blood bank in Fresno via bus.

As I had ordered it in the morning, I thought that there was ample time for the Fresno blood bank to deliver it to our local bus depot so I would receive it by noon. But noon came and went and no cryoprecipitate was delivered to the hospital. After a few frantic phone calls I realized that the package had been taken all the way to Bakersfield, the end of the line. A few more phone calls, and I was assured that it would be delivered to me by the same bus returning from Bakersfield that evening. I sat down and sweated.

By evening I received the cryoprecipitate and infused it into Peter's blood stream. That stopped the bleeding. I also consulted an orthopedic specialist. Peter's swelling gradually decreased without causing any permanent damage to his knee.

Nowadays treating hemophilia patients has become simpler. A host of commercial products are on the market such as highly purified factor VIII, porcine (swine) factor VIII, and genetically engineered varieties. They are readily available and can be easily infused. Some hospitals have designated clinics that cater to the needs of hemophilia patients. In such facilities, the child's family members are taught to give these preparations in their own homes, as needed.

A new technique involving gene therapy is being tried by Richard Sheldon's team in Cambridge, Massachusetts. His group removed skin cells from hemophilic patients and introduced into them a gene that produced factor VIII. They grew a batch of such modified cells in the laboratory and injected them into the bodies of six hemophilic patients. The cells produced factor VIII. Four of the patients thus treated needed less of their usual injections of factor VIII and had less bleeding for up to ten months. It is hoped that such techniques will eliminate the need for hemophilia patients to undergo periodic painful injections of factor VIII.

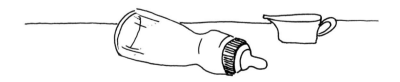

The Story of Nuclear Medicine

When I requested a nuclear scan on Lora Robinson, who had an excruciating pain over her right knee, her mother was very concerned.

"Are the radioactive dyes that you mentioned really safe?" she wanted to know.

"Of course, they are," I replied. "They emit very little radiation, which the body eliminates very rapidly. We've come a long way in safely diagnosing diseases."

It all started with a Sunday lunch in the year 1911. Gregory Hevesy, a Hungarian chemist, suspected that his landlady was compromising on the quality of some of the food items that she served. The landlady served pie on Sundays and Hevesy suspected that she mixed the leftover pieces of the pie into other food items and served them during the week. In those days, refrigeration was not readily available and leftover foods could easily get contaminated with bacteria. Whatever the reason, Hevesy wanted proof that the landlady was indeed recycling unhealthy food before confronting her. He had an ingenious idea.

Hevesy at that time was employed at Ernest Rutherford's laboratory at Cambridge, working on the separation of radioactive lead from ordinary lead; thus he had access to radioactive substances. One Sunday after lunch, when nobody was looking, Hevesy mixed a tiny bit of radioactive thorium in the leftover pie. A couple of days later, the unsuspecting landlady served a soufflé to Hevesy. With a twinkle in his eye, he brought out his electroscope; when he placed the instrument near the soufflé, it immediately recorded the presence of radioactivity. I do not know how Hevesy and the landlady got along after the confrontation, but by doing that experiment Hevesy opened the gates of radio-active tracer technique.

In 1924, Hevesy used radioactive tracers such as bismuth-210 and lead-210 to study the metabolism of animals. Later, in 1935, he used phosphorous-32 to study their metabolism. He followed the radioactive phosphorous as it entered a plant through its roots in the soil, going then into the intestines of an animal that ate the plant, and from the intestines into the animal's bones. Finally, he detected the phosphorous getting excreted in the urine. Thus, the phosphorous ended its long journey in the soil from which it originally came! For his pioneering work, Hevesy was awarded the Nobel Prize.

After the construction of nuclear reactors, many radioiso-topes became available for use in medicine. Simultaneously, sensitive instruments became available that could better detect radioactivity and quantify it accurately. One of the first organs to be examined in humans using radioactive isotopes was the thyroid gland. Thyroid function was measured by injecting ra-dioactive iodine into the blood stream and then measuring the radioactivity over the thyroid gland as the gland metabolized the iodine. Thus, hyper and hypothyroidism were detected.

Using radioisotopes, every organ in the body can be anatomi-cally visualized and its functioning measured accurately. This branch of science is called "Nuclear Medicine." Nowadays, ra-dioisotopes are used in more than 10 million *in vivo* diagnostic tests and in 100 million laboratory tests that are performed each year. These tests have alleviated great suffering and prolonged the lives of millions of people.

Lora's bone scan was normal. Next time you step into the nuclear medicine department for a thyroid scan or bone scan, remember that it all started with a pie and an unscrupulous landlady!

A Parasite From Pharaoh's Era

*B*rittney, a very pretty girl with beautiful black hair and long eyelashes, was brought to my office for dust particles stuck in her eyelashes. She also had head lice.

"I've used A-200, RID, and Nix," Brittney's mother said. "It's not helping. She still has head lice. Every day I clean her lashes and by evening she's full of these dust particles."

I examined Brittney. There were a few lice in her hair, with hundreds of white eggs scattered like stars in a dark sky. I used a magnifying glass and took a close look at her eyelashes; the dust particles turned out to be lice too. Families of them were resting at the roots of her lashes, each family the size of a small mustard seed.

Throughout history, lice have been companions to man. They existed in the era of Pharaohs and are mentioned in the Bible. Ancient Roman coins showed the various types of lice. Over the millennia, lice have become specialized, and have evolved into different kinds that live in different parts of the human body. The lice that live on the head are called *pediculosis humanus capitis*. Some live on the body and are called *pediculosis humanus corporis*. A different kind of louse specializes in living in pubic hair and is known as *phthirus pubis*. These lice look like crabs and hence are called "Crab Lice". Occasionally the crab lice, which love to wander, travel upwards and live in the hair of armpits or in eyelashes. In children, crab lice come from close contact with infested adults, especially from their mothers. That was probably how Brittney got the eyelash infestation.

A louse lives for just a month, but it lays about 150 eggs

during its lifetime. The eggs hatch in a week, mature in another week, and start laying eggs themselves; that is how lice multiply very fast. They live on blood, inject their salivary juices into the skin, and deposit fecal matter on it, causing itching, ulcers, and bacterial infections. Body lice also carry the typhus infection. Hence, it is imperative to get rid of them effectively.

I prescribed a special eye ointment for Brittney's eyelashes, which eliminated the lice there; a shampoo for the head lice was also effective.

Nowadays, lice are developing resistance to most of the common anti-lice medications. More than 100,000 cases of resistant head lice have occurred in this country in the last few years, and many children miss school because of lice infestation.

New treatments for the resistant lice are emerging. One non-pesticide product which was tried in Israel is called "Hair Clean" and is awaiting FDA approval. Some doctors treat the resistant lice with petroleum jelly, which suffocates and kills the lice; a low-tech method, certainly! Other doctors give antibiotics to affected children. When a louse sucks blood, these antibiotics eliminate the bacteria in the louse's gut, disrupt its digestive system, and kill the louse. Now there's a high-tech method for you!

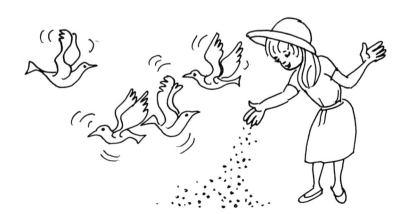

Why Is a Snake on the Medical Emblem?

A mother asked me about the significance of the snake coiled around the staff on the medical emblem. I shared with her some very interesting mythological stories about this symbol, and I'd like to share them with you as well. Since times immemorial, the snake fascinated the ancient Egyptians, Indians, Greeks, and many others; they associated it with fertility and rejuvenation, perhaps because it easily sheds its old skin for a new one, symbolizing renewal. The snake also is regarded as a protector in some Asian cultures. In India, stories are told about king cobras guarding untold treasures; and Adisesha, the snake god, is said to protect Lord Vishnu under his thousand hoods.

The ancient Greeks also believed in the healing powers of a snake, as the following story illustrates. When Glaucus, the son of King Minos, was bitten by a snake and died, the king asked his physician, Polyeidos, to revive him. Polyeidos expressed his inability to do so, and the enraged king placed him in a tomb along with his son's body, with instructions that the physician should be released only after Glaucus was brought back to life. As Polyeidos sat dejected in the tomb, a snake emerged from the darkness and approached Glaucus' body. Polyeidos promptly chopped off its head. Soon, another snake came out and, realizing that its mate had died, fetched some herbs and placed them on its spouse's body. The dead snake came to life and both of them slithered away happily. Polyeidos picked up the same herb and placed it on the body of Glaucus, who promptly came back to life.

The staff with the coiled snake in the medical symbol belonged to the Greek god Asclepius, son of the god Apollo. Both the staff and the snake conveyed the healing process and were easily interchangeable—everyone is familiar with the story of Moses changing his staff into a snake.

Asclepius learned medicine and the art of healing from a wise Centaur named Cheiron, who was a healer. Cheir in Greek means "hand"; from this, words like chirurgy (surgery) and chiropractor originated. Asclepius had many children, of whom two, Hygeia and Panakei, served in the Trojan War as surgeons. From Hygeia, who was associated with good health, we get the word "hygiene"; Panakei could cure everything, and so gave us the word "panacea".

Asclepius was an excellent physician, better than we modern ones, because he could revive the dead. When Hippolytos died, the goddess Artemus requested Asclepius to bring him back to life. Asclepius revived Hippolytos for a huge fee. Hades, the god of the dead, promptly complained to Zeus that Asclepius was cheating the kingdom of the dead. Zeus concurred that it was not nice to fool Mother Nature and dispatched Asclepius to the underworld with a thunderbolt.

Asclepius remained trapped in the underworld until the Romans, who called him "Aesculapius", sought his help during a terrible plague. Aesculapius appeared to one of the Roman envoys in a dream and told him, "Fear not, but take good heed of this snake coiled about my staff; mark it well and you may know me by it."

By and by, his snake and staff were accepted as a medical emblem, a symbol of healing and care.

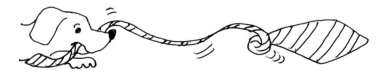

Old Medicine for a Young Heart

*J*ennifer, a cute 11-month-old girl with attractive eyes, had a stormy infant life. She was born with multiple heart defects: a narrowing of the pulmonary artery, a small right ventricle, and holes in the septum of her heart. A surgeon performed several operations on her heart to save her life. Even though the immediate danger was averted, her tired heart failed to pump enough blood into her circulation, causing a condition called "congestive heart failure" (CHF). To treat her CHF and to stimulate her heart, Jennifer was started on a drug that has been known to doctors for more than 750 years. That prompted me to review and reflect on the history of this miracle medication.

Natives around world have known for centuries that plant and animal extracts affect the heart. In Africa, strophanthus gratus vine seed extract was used as an arrow poison. Ancient Egyptians knew that squill or sea onion extract stimulates the heart; the ancient Romans used squill extract as a diuretic, heart tonic, and vermin poison. And the Chinese have for centuries used the dried skin of common toads as a heart stimulant.

Due credit, however, should be given to Dr. William Withering of Britain for scientific analysis and standardization of one of the plant extracts that have an effect on the heart. Dr. Withering was making a routine trip from his home in Birmingham to see patients in a Stafford infirmary. Midway, while the horses were being changed, Dr. Withering was asked to check on an old lady with edema. He did, and thought that the lady would die soon. A few weeks later when he inquired about her, he was told to his surprise that the old lady was alive and doing well. He was informed that the lady was given an herbal tea containing some 20 ingredients.

Dr. Withering, in addition to being a good doctor, was also a botanist and had written a book on plants. He realized that one of the ingredients in the tea the old lady consumed was an extract from a plant called foxglove. This plant had purple flowers in the shape of fingers and hence its botanical name is *digitalis purpura*. He had heard that foxglove extract had helped a few patients with edema. Dr. Withering began to experiment with foxglove extract, trying it on the poor patients of Birmingham, whom he saw for free.

After many trials he found that the extract caused increased urine output and reduced edema in some patients. He defined the types of patients who might benefit from the foxglove extract—by then called digitalis—and standardized his preparation. He further developed accurate dosage schedules based on his careful observations and warned that this highly beneficial medication, if misused, could be a potent poison. Inexperienced physicians ignored Dr. Withering's instructions and used digitalis carelessly, poisoning many patients. They blamed Dr. Withering for their mistakes and digitalis fell into disrepute. Patients who needed digitalis died because it was not given.

Another 150 years would pass before digitalis would again be recognized as a potent cardiac stimulant and a medicine useful for heartbeat irregularities. A good medicine had at last been revived! Good for Jennifer!

Nowadays we have purified digitalis called "digoxin"; we gave it to Jennifer and her heart failure came under control. The last time I saw her, she was developing normally.

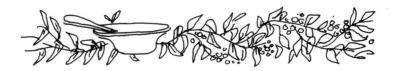

The Birth of Vitamins

"Make sure you give Cindy her vitamin drops daily," I advised Mrs. Belmont. "That's the problem, doctor; she spits the stuff out. It probably tastes awful! I wonder who discovered them!" Mrs. Belmont replied. That comment made me go to the library in search of the birth of vitamins.

In the latter half of the 19th Century, sailors in the Japanese navy were affected by a peculiar disease: they felt weak, and developed paralysis of their hands and feet; some became very ill and died. This disease was also recognized sporadically in natives of the Dutch East Indies (now Indonesia); they called it "beriberi", which meant "very weak".

Takaki, the Director General of the Japanese Navy, was concerned because one third of his sailors were sick with the disease at any given time. Being smart, he noted that British sailors and his own officers on ships did not suffer from it. He found that ordinary sailors on his ships consumed a monotonous diet of polished white rice, fish, and vegetables, whereas the British sailors (and his own officers) ate a variety of foods. Consequently, Takaki introduced a few British items like barley, meats, and evaporated milk to his sailors' diet. Like magic, beriberi virtually disappeared in the sailors. Takaki thought that supplementing extra proteins cured beriberi.

Sometimes good things go unnoticed, and Takaki's treatment for beriberi was not recognized. Beriberi was eliminated at sea, but it was endemic in the Dutch East Indies, causing the deaths of hundreds of natives every year.

Christian Eijkman, a Dutch military physician, was

investigating the cause of beriberi about that time, and noticed that the disease was prevalent in prisons. Prisoners who ate polished rice developed beriberi and those who consumed crude rice did not. Eijkman surmised that a germ or toxin in the polished rice was responsible for beriberi, and that the crude unpolished rice had an antidote to the germ or poison.

With these thoughts in mind, Eijkman, who was then employed as a bacteriologist in a hospital, tried to infect a few chickens with the presumed germ or toxin from beriberi patients. When the chickens did not develop beriberi for a long time, Eijkman was disappointed. However, one day in 1896, his chickens developed weakness and paralysis. Eijkman thought that he could finally transmit the disease and proceeded to isolate the germ, but however much he tried, he could not isolate it from the sick chickens. While he was still involved with his experiments, the chickens suddenly recovered from the illness and became healthy, leaving Eijkman very puzzled.

Like a good detective, Eijkman started questioning the hospital staff and the cooks who fed the chickens. He found that hospital cooks changed frequently. One cook fed the chickens scraps from hospital patients' food, which consisted mainly of polished rice. It was during this period that the chickens developed paralysis. Another cook, deciding that the chickens did not deserve polished rice that was meant for humans, gave them unpolished rice with husks. During this period, the chickens recovered.

Eijkman realized that beriberi was not due to a toxin or germ; rather, the polished rice was deficient in a factor that prevented beriberi. For the first time, it was recognized that a lack of minute amounts of a certain factor could cause a serious disease. (The scientists Jansen and Donath established much later that this factor was thiamine.) For his pioneering work, Eijkman was awarded a Nobel Prize in 1929.

Casimer Funk, a Polish biochemist working in London in 1911, isolated a substance that he thought was a beriberi-preventing factor. What he discovered was nicotinic acid. This substance had a chemical structure with a nitrogen atom and two hydrogen atoms (-NH2), the so-called amine group at one end. Because this trace substance was essential for life, he named it vitamine (life-amine). Later it was found that a few of these trace substances did not possess an amine group. Thus the name vitamine was a misnomer.

In 1920, Jack Drummond, an English biochemist, suggested the terminal "e" be dropped; these essential substances then came to be called vitamins.

So the next time you give your child vitamin drops, or pop in a vitamin pill, remember that it all started with sailors and chickens!

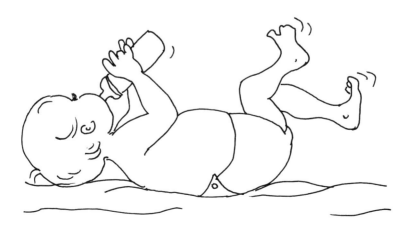

Chance and a Prepared Mind

*G*inger, 15 years old, had a streptococcal sore throat for which I prescribed penicillin.

"Ginger, who discovered penicillin?" I asked as she was leaving my office.

"Fleming, I guess," she replied.

Almost everyone knows who discovered penicillin, and how. But many are unaware of the chance occurrences and coincidences that led to its discovery.

Alexander Fleming, a London bacteriologist who had the habit of saving everything, because he thought he could use it later, had in the summer of 1928 saved several culture plates of staphylococci long after he needed them for his experiments. Finally, one day, he threw them in a dish that was scantily filled with a disinfectant. Only a few culture plates got immersed, leaving the top ones intact. When a fellow-scientist stopped by to check on the research, Fleming picked up a culture plate at random from the disinfectant tray. In showing it to his colleague, he noticed that colonies of bacteria known as staphylococci were not growing around a large colony of a fungus (or mold) that had accidentally contaminated the plate. On this chance observation, Fleming surmised that the mold secreted a substance that disintegrated the bacteria, a process called lysis, and killed them. The mold belonged to the genus penicillium, and hence Fleming named the substance that killed the bacteria "penicillin".

If Fleming had not picked that particular plate, or if that plate had fallen into the disinfectant, he would have missed the chance to discover penicillin.

Another mystery: When scientists inoculated staphylococci

and the mold on the culture plate simultaneously, the mold failed to lyse the bacteria. This was because the bacteria grew faster than the mold at temperatures above 70 F, and not enough mold grew to produce adequate quantities of penicillin to kill the bacteria. When scientists inoculated the culture plates with the mold first, to allow it to grow bigger, and later inoculated the plate with bacteria, they noticed lysis. How was it that in Fleming's famous culture plate the mold grew big, even though the fungal spore must have contaminated the plate at the same time he was seeding it with staphylococci?

In the summer months of July and August 1928, a cold wave engulfed London for nine days. Fleming's lab was not well insulated and temperatures fell below 68 F. In colder conditions, molds grow faster than bacteria. Thus, Fleming's mold had a head start! By the time the staphylococci slowly grew, enough mold was present to produce penicillin that caused lysis of bacteria around the mold. Without that cold wave, the mold would have grown more slowly and no lysis of bacteria would have occurred.

In spite of all these coincidences, ordinary people would have missed the bacterial lysis around the mold, or not realized its significance. Even some of Fleming's colleagues did not think much of it at that time, but Fleming eventually was awarded the Nobel Prize for his discovery. The more original a finding, the more obvious it seems afterward; but only a prepared mind can grab a chance when one comes along!

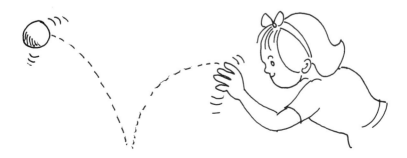

The Story of Epilepsy

Mrs. Maples, Lisa's mother, was happily partici-
pating in the three-year-old's make-believe
games, when the child suddenly rolled her eyes
upward and fell back unconscious. Lisa stiffened for a few seconds—to Mrs. Maples it seemed like hours—and violently shook
her arms and legs. Mrs. Maples, unable to stop the seizures, panicked and called an ambulance. She had barely hung up the phone
when Lisa stopped shaking and became limp. By the time the
ambulance had arrived, Lisa was able to recognize her mother
and speak a few words, although groggy.

Lisa had an attack of tonic-clonic seizures, commonly called
"epilepsy". Epilepsy has been well known for centuries and has
been described in a Babylonian medical text dating from around
650 BC. It was known as a "sacred disease" or "falling sickness".
Egyptians and Romans were aware of it. They believed that evil
spirits and demons possessed the affected person.

Treatment of epilepsy has varied over the centuries. In Egypt,
only the rich could afford treatment. The patients were brought
to a temple where the priests conducted elaborate ceremonies
with strange incantations, invoking the various gods who were
protecting the patient to scare away the demon. Often, the priest
would dress like a powerful god and appear in front of the patient to frighten the evil spirit away. Over the years, herbs, oint-
ments, precious stones, and vegetables believed to have magical
properties were added to treat epilepsy along with strange incantations.

In Greece, too, epilepsy and mental disorders were viewed as
demonic or divine visitations. Displeased gods would send the

disease to punish people who had erred. The patients were treated in shrines by mystical incantations. Patients were allowed to sleep in the temples. An attendant would dress up as a god and would walk slowly among the patients in the dark, compassionately touching the suffering ones; the patients, confused and ailing, would believe that a god had indeed visited them and felt they might get better. If a patient improved, the priests took credit for it; if not, the priests discharged the poor man from the shrine, proclaiming that since the gods were displeased with him no improvement was noticed.

Some Romans drank the warm blood of freshly slain gladiators as a cure for epilepsy. Much later, Peter of Spain, a physician of the 13th Century, advised seizure patients to consume the liver of vultures for nine days or the gallbladder of a freshly killed dog at the moment of the seizure. Eventually, Peter became Pope John XXI.

Medical practice in colonial America was not far behind in unusual treatments for epilepsy. Barbers, clergymen, civil officers, and plantation owners treated diseases without any hesitation. The treatments were amusing and sometimes perhaps dangerous. Mithridate (dogtooth-violet plant) extracts, antimonial cup, and oriental bezoar stone were used to treat many diseases including epilepsy. Bezoars are stones found in the stomach and intestines that are believed to have magical properties. A "Spirit of Skull" treatment was offered specifically for epilepsy. Moss from an excavated skull of a man who had died of a violent cause was mixed with wine and several other ingredients to make the "spirit of skull". It is interesting to note that one of the last medications given to King Charles II of England on his deathbed was 30 drops of "spirit of skull".

In colonial days in America, another treatment called *confectio antiepileptica* required a minimum of three pulverized human skulls of men who had died violently; the powder was mixed with several liquids. Other remedies consisted of pulverized human hearts, brains of young men who had died under the age of 24, and human blood.

John Winthrop, Jr., governor of Connecticut Colony and Fellow of the Royal Society of London for Improving of Natural Knowledge, mixed alchemy, astrology, and other mystical sciences to treat ailments. He had a great reputation as a physician. One of his sure cures was recorded thus: "Clip the patient's nails when the fever is coming on. Put the nail clippings in a fine linen bag. Tie the bag above a live eel's neck in a tub of water. The eel will die and the patient will recover." In addition, bleeding and purging treatments were sometimes given for epilepsy.

I did not have to search for skulls or eels to treat Lisa. After proper investigation, I started her on Phenobarbital, which controlled her seizures. The last I saw Lisa, she was doing fine.

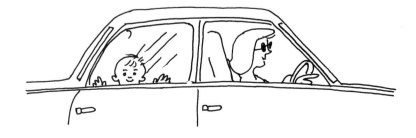

Napoleon's Itch

*S*teven, six months old, was brought to my office because of sleeplessness. He was very uncomfortable, especially at night. There was no obvious cause for Steven's sleeplessness: no history of a fever, a cold, or a cough; nor was his mother giving him any caffeine containing beverages.

During the examination, I noticed a red rash over Steven's abdomen, back, hands, and face. The rash was probably itching and poor Steven was trying his best to scratch with his tiny fingers, leaving a few marks here and there.

I inquired further. Steven was not on any medications. He was not allergic to milk formula, and his mother was not trying new body soaps or lotions or new clothes, especially any made out of wool. There were no pets in the house.

"Do you have a rash or an itch?" I asked Steven's mother.

"Yes," she replied.

With her permission I examined her hands and finger webs. There were pinpoint red spots over her finger webs with multiple scratch marks. On further questioning, I learned that Steven's father also had similar itchy lesions. Now the diagnosis became very obvious in Steven. The whole family had a disease called scabies.

In adults and older children, scabies is usually seen as small red spots that itch intensely. Face, neck, palms, and soles are spared. In infants, the lesions look different and all parts of the body are affected, including the face. Because of the itching, children don't sleep well. The scratches may get infected or eczema may develop.

Scabies is a very common childhood infection caused by a

parasitic mite called sarcoptes scabiei, and is transmitted by direct contact with an infected person. Occasionally, it is transmitted from dogs and is called canine scabies. Avian mites from chickens can also cause skin lesions. The parasite burrows into the skin and lays eggs and the body reacts to the mite antigens by producing an intense itch.

As I was reviewing the literature, I came across an interesting fact about Napoleon Bonaparte, who suffered from an intense itch for a long time. There were many causes for Napoleon's itch. He suffered from gastritis, which in those days was treated with an antacid preparation containing arsenic; arsenic was found in Napoleon's skin, and could have caused the itching. The physician Antommarchi, who conducted an autopsy on the emperor, noted skin lesions resembling a disease called dermatitis herpetiformis, which could have caused the itching, but there is yet another explanation for Napoleon's itch. In those days, scabies was rampant throughout the French Army. At one time 400,000 men, including many officers, suffered from the disease, and Napoleon could very easily have contracted the disease from them. Jean-Nicholas Corvisart, Napoleon's physician, treated Napoleon with sulfur baths, which until recently was a treatment for scabies. It thus seems very likely that Napoleon suffered from scabies.

The medicine I prescribed for Steven cured the infection, but every time I see someone scratching with scabies, I remember Napoleon's itch.

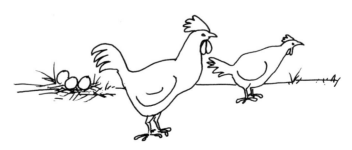

Listen, But Don't Touch!
Story of the First Stethoscope

When I was in my second year of medical school, I envied those seniors who walked leisurely through the medical wards, casually dangling their stethoscopes. They flocked around a patient, took turns examining him, and whispered mysteriously the secrets they unearthed from his bowels or his chest with their stethoscopes.

No other instrument identifies a doctor so unequivocally. Who invented this status symbol? The credit goes to a puny French physician, Rene Laennec. Laennec was short—just five feet three inches tall—and had blue eyes and chestnut hair. He had a big prominent forehead and high cheekbones, all of which made him unforgettable once someone had seen him.

Laennec was a brilliant doctor and researcher. In 1802, he described the narrowing of one of the heart valves, a condition called mitral stenosis. He also discovered the significance of a membrane called the peritoneum that lined various organs in the abdomen. He recognized an infection of the peritoneum called peritonitis and described the changes that occur as a result of the infection. He studied tuberculosis and documented its effect on the peritoneal membrane. While studying the peritoneum, Laennec noticed scarring of the livers of alcoholics and the peculiar dark yellow color they exhibited. In Greek, a tawny tint is known as kirrhos; from this came the word cirrhosis of the liver. Liver damage caused by alcohol is called Laennec's cirrhosis. Laennec conducted all this research while he was still a medical student!

Many years later, while employed as a physician at Necker Hospital in Paris, he needed to examine a young woman with heart disease. Because of the sex and age of the patient he could not apply his ear directly to her chest to hear the heart sounds. He was in a fix.

The story goes that Laennec was out walking alone when he saw some boys playing with a long piece of wood. One boy put his ear to one end of the stick to hear the scratching sounds the other boy made at the other end. Laennec knew that some hollow objects conducted sounds better. Back in the hospital, he rolled a quire of paper into a cylinder and applied one end to the chest of the young woman and the other end to his ear. Lo and behold, he heard the heart and breath sounds very clearly. The stethoscope was invented!

By using his device Laennec described various kinds of breath sounds, such as wheezing and rales, to name a couple. When a patient died, he noted the pathology in the heart or the lungs that had caused the murmur or the peculiar breath sound. Soon, he was able to diagnose many lung conditions just by listening to his patient's chest with his gadget.

Laennec called his invention a stethoscope (stethos means chest and skopos means observer). Sometimes, he called it "le cilindre". He manufactured his stethoscopes in two small segments that could be attached before using, and could be carried in a coat pocket or inside a top hat.

Nowadays, stethoscopes come in various sizes and colors with one head, two heads, or even three heads; one even has a watch on one side of it. It seems as if the stethoscope has become part and parcel of a doctor's body; without it one is not a physician, just as without a trunk there is no elephant!

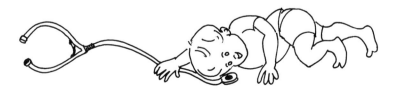

Juvenile Rheumatoid Arthritis?
Rare, But It Happens!

April and June are sisters, born six years apart. When April, the elder, was fifteen months old, her parents brought her to my office because she was eating poorly. A typical day's eating consisted of two ounces of milk, four ounces of juice, and some cereal and pieces of fruit.

April was sick-looking, irritable, peevish, and tired. A normal child more or less doubles her birth weight by the age of five months, and triples it at twelve months. April's birth weight was six pounds and six ounces. She should have weighed nineteen pounds by her first birthday. At fifteen months, for her height, her weight should have been at least twenty-one pounds, but she weighed only seventeen-and-a-half. April did not have any problem with swallowing nor was there any obvious evidence of a disease that precluded normal eating. Except for her being grossly underweight, April's initial examination was normal.

A child whose weight is below the fifth percentile in children's growth charts, or a weight that is 20 percent below the ideal weight, is said to have a condition called "Failure to Thrive." One of the main causes, as was evident in April, is inadequate food intake. April's parents had been counseled about child nutrition and were well aware of how much to feed her. They were very caring and loved her; there was no evidence of child neglect.

Preliminary laboratory tests did not show any evidence of a metabolic or hormonal disease. But I found April to be slightly anemic and started her on iron therapy.

A simple age-old test called Erythrocyte Sedimentation Rate (ESR) consists of placing a cubic milliliter of blood in a standardized glass tube and measuring the length of fall of the red cell column in an hour. Normal children have an ESR of 4 to 20 millimeters per hour; if the ESR is higher, it signifies an active disease process in the body. April's ESR was 57 millimeters; what active disease could be lurking within her?

In medicine, the saying goes that the number of tests ordered is directly proportional to the degree of ignorance about the diagnosis. After consulting experts, I ordered a battery of tests on April to cover both common and uncommon diseases. This time, too, all the tests were reported normal except a urine culture that grew a germ called E. Coli. Recurrent urinary infections could cause failure to thrive. I shouted "Eureka" and treated April with appropriate antibiotics, following through with necessary X rays and tests to find any anatomical abnormalities of the urinary system. There were none. But April still refused to eat and her weight did not budge up even a single ounce. We were back to square one.

One day, April herself revealed the diagnosis to me. She cried, complained of pain in her ankle and knee joints, and did not want to be moved. I did not find much swelling or redness of the joints, but my examination must have caused so much pain that even my entering the room during the subsequent visits made her cry uncontrollably. Her parents recalled that she had complained of occasional leg pains.

A child failing to thrive, with painful joints—after excluding infectious causes—is likely to have a disease called Juvenile Rheumatoid Arthritis (JRA). Certain tests such as rheumatoid factor, and antinuclear antibody tests, will clinch the diagnosis of JRA when results are positive. They were all negative. Since in many cases these tests do come out negative even when the patient has JRA, I decided to treat her for the disease. If April improved, then she must have had the disease. After consulting a specialist I started April on an appropriate dose of good old baby aspirin.

It worked like magic. Her joint pains subsided, and her appetite came back to some extent; however, she still needed to be tube-fed for proper nutrition. She started gaining weight. Her parents had poor compliance in giving her aspirin every four hours; hence she was switched to another medication called Naprosyn. As JRA could affect the eyes, causing a condition called iridocyclitis, her eyes were examined periodically and they were normal. She was given physical therapy to lessen the stiffness of her joints. The last time I saw April, she was in fourth grade and was doing well. Her weight had eventually stabilized at the lower limits of normal; however, she continued to need Naprosyn to control her symptoms.

Remember April's sister June? June was six years younger than April, and at about the age of twenty months she too failed to gain weight, complained of leg pains, was anemic, and her ESR was elevated. You know the diagnosis, don't you? After appropriate consultation, I started June on Naprosyn; that greatly helped to alleviate the joint pains. Her antinuclear antibody test was positive, favoring the diagnosis of JRA.

April and June, two sisters, presented with the same rare disease, at almost the same age. It's odd, isn't it?

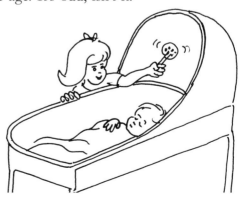

Acne That Wasn't Acne

I have known Mark since he was six years old. He was cute and had very pleasant manners. At about the age of nine, Mark developed seizures, which scared his mother. After proper investigations and a consultation with a neurologist, Mark was started on a medication to control his seizures. But because the seizures still were poorly controlled, he was started on another medication, and after a few weeks, a third drug was added to the regimen.

Unfortunately, Mark continued to have two to three seizures a month. In spite of all this, Mark did well in school.

Taking a good medical history, which includes a family history, often paves the way to arriving at a correct diagnosis. Findings such as a small white spot on the skin may appear unimportant, but once the diagnosis becomes obvious all the seemingly unimportant findings fit together like a puzzle.

Mark had white skin patches over his arms, legs, and back. His mother had small white spots on her skin; his maternal grandmother also had white spots. Mark's uncle suffered from seizures; so did his mother's uncle.

When Mark was 14 years old, he developed minimal acne on the face. He told me, later, that he tried an ointment that was available over the counter, but it produced no improvement.

Stubborn seizures, acne-like lesions, white spots, a family history of seizures—these, when taken together, pointed to a disease called "tuberous sclerosis", a hereditary disorder with variable degrees of developmental delay, seizures, and peculiar skin lesions. It is inherited as a dominant disease; 50 percent of the children born to an affected parent are likely to have it.

The acne-like lesions that Mark had on his face were not acne at all, but characteristic lesions of tuberous sclerosis called *adenoma sebaceum*. Children with the disease have thickened nodular swellings in the brain, which can be seen in a CAT scan. In fact, Mark had a small lesion in his brain. Doctors believe that these abnormally thickened areas in the brain cause seizures and developmental problems. While people with mild involvement can lead full, productive lives, severely affected persons may need to be institutionalized.

The last time I saw Mark, multiple specialists were involved in his care, and he was doing well. He had a girlfriend and the genetic specialist had cautioned him that if he had children, half of them were likely to get the disease. His seizures were well controlled with various medications. Mark knew all the possible complications and hurdles that lay ahead in his life's journey, and was ready to face them, optimistic and cheerful as ever.

Life is like a football game. Mark was ready to tackle his problems, block his fears, and push forward with dogged determination.

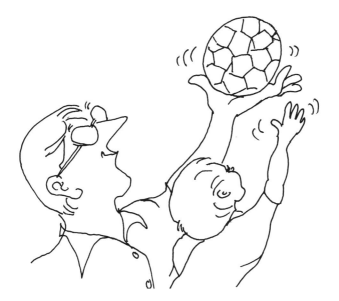

Blue Boy's Story

*J*ohn was a charming two-year-old when I first came to know him. The most striking feature about him was his skin: it was dusky blue-gray in color and his lips were blue. He had a loud heart murmur. John would become breathless after taking a few steps and would tire easily. Needless to say, he had a serious problem.

To understand what John had, some knowledge of the anatomy of the heart and circulation is necessary. The human heart is an incredible pump with four chambers. The upper chambers are called the atria and the lower ones the ventricles. Deoxygenated blue blood from the peripheral parts of the body drains first into the right atrium, and then into the right ventricle, which pumps the blood via the pulmonary artery into the lungs. There, the blood gets oxygenated, becomes red and drains into the left atrium via pulmonary veins. From there it passes into the left ventricle, which pumps the blood via the aorta into various parts of the body. The right and left sides of the heart are separate and blood does not get mixed between the two sides. However, even though the sides are separate, they pump in unison 72 times a minute, about 2,877 million beats in one's lifetime. Indeed an amazing performance!

John had four congenital malformations in his heart: the pulmonary artery was narrowed and tight; there was a hole between the left and right ventricles; the aorta was shifted to the right and originated from both ventricles; and the right ventricular wall was very thickened. John had a condition called the "tetralogy of Fallot".

Why the name? In about 1761, a Dutch physician called

Edward Sandifort described a blue boy who became increasingly breathless and died at the age of 12. At the autopsy, Dr. Sandifort noticed several malformations in the boy's heart. However, a full century elapsed before the four cardiac abnormalities we observed in John were first recognized in another patient by a professor of anatomical pathology in Marseilles, France. A group of four is called a tetralogy, and since the discoverer was a Dr. Etienne-Louis Fallot, this condition is named after him.

In John, the deoxygenated blue blood returning from the various parts of his body never reached the lungs for oxygenation because of the narrowing of the pulmonary artery. Instead, most of the blood passed through the hole between the ventricles, short-circuiting the lungs, and was pumped back to various parts of the body. This explained why John's skin was gray-blue and his lips were deep blue. As John grew up, his body needed more oxygen, which his heart could not deliver. Hence, he was breathless after taking a few steps.

John was referred to a nearby children's hospital, where he underwent surgery. The hole in the ventricular septum was closed with a Teflon patch and the pulmonary artery was repaired. He did well post-operatively.

At the age of four John was healthy. He looked pink and his blue color had vanished. As usual, he was full of smiles.

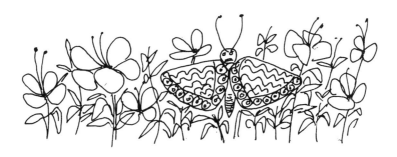

A Disease of Mirror Image

I have known Tracy since she was two months old. During a routine physical examination, I noticed that her heart sounds, instead of being more prominent over the left side, were better heard over the right side of her chest. That was unusual.

As she grew, Tracy developed a cough and wheezed. A diagnosis of bronchitis with asthma was made and she was treated with antibiotics and medications that dilate the bronchi, the branches of the windpipe. Tracy improved. However, her cough continued and she needed bronchodilators constantly.

When Tracy was five years old, I suspected she had a sinus infection. An X ray of the sinuses showed haziness and fluid in ethmoid, sphenoid, and maxillary sinuses, suggesting a chronic infection. She was treated with antibiotics intermittently. At seven years of age, Tracy had a chest X ray, which showed a mild dilatation of bronchi in her lungs, a condition called bronchiectasis.

Investigations over the years had revealed that Tracy's heart was located over the right side of her chest, a condition called "dextrocardia". That was why I could hear the heart sounds better on the right side of her chest. In addition, the liver, which is normally on the right side of the abdomen, was on the left side, and her stomach and spleen, which are normally on the left, were on the right. In summary, the organs that are on the right were moved to the left side and vice versa, a mirror image translocation. This condition is called *situs inversus*. Very strange indeed!

Intestines, bronchi, middle ear, sinuses, and other organs are lined with cells that have small hair-like projections called cilia. There are 275 cilia per cell and they move synchronously 7 to

22 times per second. On the cells lining the human respiratory tract, a huge number of cilia (1,000,000,000/cm. squared) are involved in sweeping mucus and other particles such as dust and dead cells. If the cilia are absent or don't function properly, secretions and bacteria accumulate in the lungs, middle ear, and other organs, causing recurrent infections. Moreover, in very early embryonic development, it is believed that gut cells need cilia to migrate properly so that other organs like the liver and spleen move into proper positions. If the intestines don't move properly, other organs fall into abnormal positions. That was why Tracy had situs inversus and recurrent infections.

The combination of sinus infection, situs inversus, bronchiectasis, and decreased fertility (in males) is called Kartegener's syndrome or primary ciliary dyskinesia. Tracy probably had dysfunctional cilia, which did not clear her secretions effectively. That led to the various problems mentioned earlier.

The last time I saw Tracy, her infections and respiratory problems were under control. However, she will continue to have those problems, and will need medications on a long-term basis.

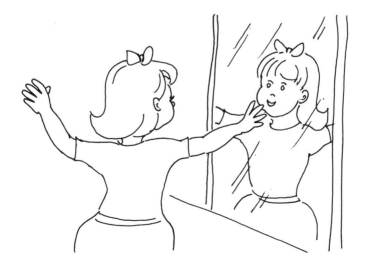

An Odd Reason for Hives

Twelve-year-old Vanessa came to my office with hives all over her body. The rash was itching and I gave her an antihistamine. Vanessa also had a sinus infection that I treated with an antibiotic.

Vanessa came back in a week. Her rash was almost gone and the itching had subsided. I learned that she had had this rash off and on for several months. She was not allergic to medications or foods and there were no pets in her house. She used Dove body soap for a long time without any problems. On further questioning, I learned that Vanessa's skin rash usually appeared after a walk in cold weather, and that exposure to cool air from an air-conditioner also caused hives. Since cold temperature bothered her, Vanessa was quick to warm herself after showers.

I did a few tests, and found that a protein called immune globulin E was elevated in her blood. This indicated an allergy, so I consulted an allergy specialist who did a simple test. He placed an ice cube on Vanessa's skin, and soon she developed hives in that area. Vanessa had a condition called "cold-induced urticaria".

Many conditions can cause hives, including physical agents such as cold, heat, sunlight, and minor injury. Out of these physical agents, cold causes hives most frequently. The rash usually develops over the body parts exposed to the cold. After a shower, the skin becomes cold due to the evaporation of water and that was how Vanessa developed hives. Swimming in cold water could become dangerous for people with cold-induced urticaria; if they are very sensitive to the cold, they may develop skin puffiness, a runny nose, nasal stuffiness, and asthma.

There is no treatment for this disease except to avoid exposure to the cold. Antihistamines sometimes help. Vanessa understood her problem and avoided situations that could lead to cold
exposure. As far as I know, she has been doing well.

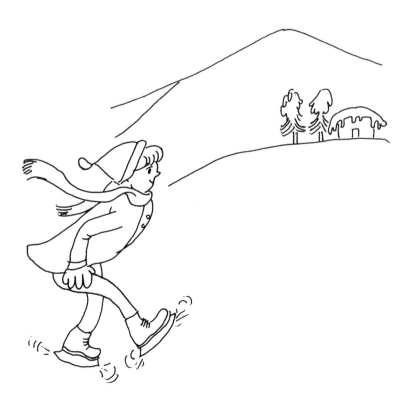

The Mother of All Rashes

*F*our-year-old Tim came to me with a patchy rash all over his body. He had a high fever that lasted ten days. He had been to the emergency room a couple of times and antibiotics were prescribed. Because there was no improvement, he was admitted to a local hospital and treated with intravenous medications and aspirin. He felt better and his mother brought him to me for a follow-up.

When I examined Tim, he looked miserable, had a mild sore throat, chaffed lips, and bloodshot eyes. A patchy purple-red rash had spread all over his body; skin was peeling off his abdomen, palms, and soles. He rubbed a little and a small patch of skin came off his fingertips. I hadn't seen such a severe rash in years; surely this must be the "mother of all rashes"!

Rashes are very common in children; they are mostly due to allergies, drugs and viral or bacterial infections. A good analysis of the patient's history and a few simple laboratory tests will often reveal the diagnosis. Tim's tests showed no evidence of bacterial infection. The way the rash developed and persisted ruled out many common causes of rash in children. What was Tim's problem then?

Tim had a very rare condition called the Kawasaki syndrome; nobody knows exactly what causes it. In 1974, Dr. Kawasaki described several children with prolonged fever, inflamed eyes, rash over their lips, hands, feet, and trunk, and enlarged lymph glands. In addition, their hearts, joints, and other parts of the body were sometimes damaged.

Because the heart condition could be serious, I referred Tim to a cardiologist, who did a test called echocardiography, an elegant noninvasive method to study the condition of the heart. Tim had developed an abnormal enlargement, or aneurysm, of the blood vessels of his heart. This could form a nidus for a blood clot and could lead to many serious complications. To prevent this mishap, we began giving him baby aspirins.

Tim improved gradually; it took about five weeks for the rash to disappear completely. Luckily, he didn't have any complications of the heart, even though it took three long years for the aneurysm to subside. Since then, as far as I know, Tim has been doing well.

Not all rashes are simple; some diseases with rashes can cause serious problems. If your child has a persistent rash with fever, please consult your doctor.

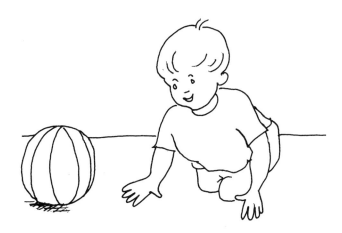

Anita's Alternate Day Fever

*A*nita Patel, ten years old, spiked a fever for five days. Peculiarly, the fever appeared only on alternate days. Anita would experience chills, shake vigorously, curl up and lie down in a fetal position. Her temperature would rise up to 105 F. In a short time Anita would sweat, her fever would come down to normal, and she would feel well again.

Anita lost her appetite with the onset of the fever. Because she got dehydrated, I admitted her into a hospital, did appropriate tests, and gave her intravenous fluids. Her parents told me that they had traveled to India a few weeks earlier. Malaria was, and still is, present in certain parts of India, and it causes intermittent fevers like Anita's. Knowing this, I went to the lab to examine a specially prepared blood smear. Under the microscope, I had no problem in identifying the malarial parasite nestled in rosettes in Anita's red blood cells. It was indeed malaria that she had, and I started her on an appropriate antimalarial drug.

The life cycle of the malarial parasite is very interesting. When a female mosquito of the anopheles species sucks blood from a malaria patient, the male and female forms of the parasite, called gametes, enter the stomach of the mosquito. The male and female gametes fuse—surprisingly they can't do this in a human—and later by a series of transformations become what are called sporozoites. They migrate to the salivary gland of the mosquito and wait patiently. When this mosquito bites another human, the sporozoites enter the human blood stream, travel to the liver and develop further to form small round bodies called merozoites that reenter the blood stream and infect thousands of red blood cells.

The merozoites multiply, and devour and rupture the red

blood cells every 24 to 48 hours depending on the species of the parasite. The remnants of the broken red cells are let out into the blood stream every 24 to 48 hours causing a high fever that is characteristic of malaria. Because the red cells are destroyed in the thousands, the person becomes anemic. Some of the merozoites miraculously develop into male and female gametes and await an anopheles mosquito bite for further development. Without a mosquito, the malarial parasite would become extinct. What a complicated life cycle!

Malaria is a major global problem occurring in more than 100 countries in Africa, Asia, and South America. More than 300 million people suffer from it; one million, mostly infants and children, die annually. In the United States, most of those affected are immigrants, visitors, or travelers returning from countries endemic with malaria.

Even though effective drugs are being used against malaria, the parasite is developing a resistance to them. Even the mosquitoes have become resistant to insecticides. A vaccine was developed for malaria, but its efficacy is not promising. Recently, scientists have developed a genetic technique of breeding altered anopheles mosquitoes that are incapable of hosting the malarial parasite. They plan to release these mosquitoes in endemic areas to replace the malaria-carrying mosquitoes. This is a very novel concept, which perhaps can be applied to other diseases that are transmitted by insects.

I advised Anita's parents to take a medication for malaria prophylaxis whenever they travel to India. Anita recovered completely without complications and went home.

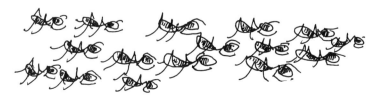

An Accidental Discovery

I saw Paul soon after birth, a cute little boy full of energy. While examining him Paul's mother asked, "Dr. Rao, his dad has cysts in his kidneys. Do you think Paul can inherit the cysts? Can you run any tests to find this out?"

Paul's blood test results showed that his kidney functions were normal. However, his ultrasound showed a slight enlargement of his kidneys, a condition called hydronephrosis. There were no cysts, but hydronephrosis is not normal. Perhaps Paul had a slight obstruction to the flow of urine; if so, the urine would back up causing an enlargement of the urinary tract, just like a thin rubber tube that swells up when the flow of water is obstructed at the other end. If there was an obstruction to Paul's urinary tract, it would need to be corrected promptly, or permanent damage would occur to his kidneys. I referred Paul to a kidney specialist.

The specialist ordered tests to find out whether the urine backed upwards from Paul's bladder when he voided. This is called a vesico-ureteral reflux, a condition that could lead to many complications. Luckily for Paul, the tests were normal. His electrolytes, blood urea nitrogen (BUN), and creatinine—substances that measure the kidney functions—were normal.

All this was good news.

When Paul was six months old, we repeated the ultrasound. At this time, there was no evidence of hydronephrosis in his kidneys. Perhaps there was a transient, partial obstruction to the flow of urine that had caused the hydronephrosis. Anyway, Paul did well.

Because Paul's dad had cysts in his kidneys, a condition called polycystic kidneys that can be inherited in an autosomal dominant manner, we investigated his family members. People with polycystic kidneys may suffer from high blood pressure, heart problems, and kidney failure. They can have cysts in their liver and pancreas, and sometimes aneurysms in the brain. Paul's paternal grandmother had an abnormal ultrasound, suggestive of kidney involvement.

"How did the doctors diagnose your husband's polycystic kidneys, when he didn't have any symptoms or signs?" I asked Paul's mother one day. I was curious.

"My husband was in an auto-accident a few months ago," she replied. "The abdominal scans done at that time showed the cysts in his kidneys. You see, Dr. Rao, it was truly an accidental discovery!"

Even though Paul is all right, polycystic kidney disease may show up later in his life; there is a 50 percent chance that this could happen. Unfortunately, at present we have no test that will diagnose the condition early. I plan to follow him closely by measuring his kidney function and performing renal ultrasounds. Time will tell.

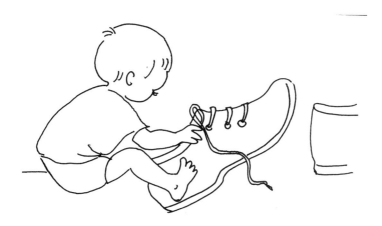

Mystery of the Half-Opened Eye

hree-year-old Matthew's mother brought him to my office with a peculiar problem—he had been unable to close his left eye for the past three days; more, when he cried, only the right side of his mouth moved. Matthew's mother told me that he had a sore throat two weeks prior to the onset of the problem. There was no history of injury to his eye or head, and there was no ear infection. Matthew was not on any medications.

I examined Matthew thoroughly. He was very cooperative. Even though he appeared normal, he could not do several things. He could not wrinkle his forehead on the left side. The right side was normal. He could not close his left eye completely. However much he tried, his eye remained half-opened. The nasolabial fold—a fold of skin between the nose and the cheek—was absent on the left side of his face. The cheek muscles were weak on the same side. When he smiled, his mouth deviated towards the right side. The rest of Matthew's physical examination was normal.

The combination of these signs pointed to paralysis of Matthew's face on the left side, a syndrome called Bell palsy, caused by an infection of, or damage to, the facial nerve. The incidence rate is about 23 per 100,000 annually. It happens suddenly, usually without any cause. Occasionally, there is a history of an ear infection, or a herpes zoster infection (shingles). Exposure to cold weather may precipitate this condition. The facial weakness appears rather suddenly in a few hours; usually, someone notices the facial asymmetry or drooling of food from one side of the mouth while eating. In addition to the signs noticed in Matthew, children with Bell palsy may have loss of taste on the affected side. Occasionally, due to the paralysis of the nerve to the middle ear, children may have abnormal sensitivity to hearing. Even ordinary conversation may seem loud. This is called hyperacusis.

Bell palsy can be caused by many medical conditions. Tumors of the brain, skull fractures, mastoid and ear infections, and demyelinating diseases can all cause Bell palsy. I requested a CAT scan of the brain to rule out some of these conditions, and the CAT scan was normal.

I started Matthew on corticosteroids, which relieve inflammation and reduce edema. As he could not blink, his left eye was dry. Hence I gave him sterile lubricant eye drops to keep the eye wet.

Matthew showed slight improvement within a week. Children with Bell palsy who show early improvement usually recover completely. When I checked Matthew in a month, he could close his left eye tight like an oyster and could smile his million-dollar smile without deviation of the mouth!

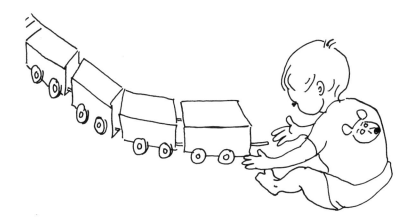

The Dog That Did Not Bark

*D*r. Watson was puzzled. "Is there any point to which you would wish to draw my attention?" he asked Sherlock Holmes.

"To the curious incident of the dog in the nighttime," the great detective replied.

"The dog did nothing in the nighttime," Watson said.

"That was the curious incident," said Sherlock.

The dog that did not bark drew the famous detective's attention in the story, "Silver Blaze." For physicians, a negative laboratory test is sometimes equally noteworthy, as the following story illustrates.

Mandy, a seven-year-old, was admitted early in the morning to a hospital with a fever of 101.9 and pain in the right wrist and left ankle. The pain had started one day earlier. Her wrist was slightly swollen, red, and felt warm and tender to the touch. Mandy winced because any movement to the wrist caused severe pain. Apart from the joint involvement and fever, the rest of her examination was normal.

Several diseases occur the way Mandy's did. An infection in the joint, called septic arthritis, or infection in the bone, called osteomyelitis, were good possibilities. Other conditions, such as rheumatic fever that follows streptococcal infections, rheumatoid arthritis, and lupus can cause joint pains and fever as well. A disease called gout, which is very rare in children, can also cause the same symptoms, but usually affects smaller joints.

After requesting appropriate blood tests and X rays, I started Mandy on an antibiotic to treat a suspected joint or bone infection.

By midday, some of the laboratory test results became available. X rays of the joints were normal. Tests for rheumatoid arthritis, gout, and past streptococcal infections were negative. A blood test called a CBC showed a total white cell count of 12,200, out of which 86 percent were lymphocytes and 10 percent were neutrophils. In an acute infection such as septic arthritis, the lymphocyte count will be low and the neutrophil count will usually be high. In Mandy, the neutrophils were very low.

Failure of the dog to bark aroused Sherlock Holmes' curiosity; failure of the neutrophils to increase in a seemingly acute infection aroused mine.

I went to the lab, checked the blood smear, and found a few very immature lymphocytes suggestive of leukemia. A bone marrow examination confirmed that Mandy had acute lymphoblastic leukemia. In children with leukemia, joints are sometimes involved in ways that may mimic an acute infection.

Mandy did well on chemotherapy and radiation, and was cancer free when she moved out of Porterville.

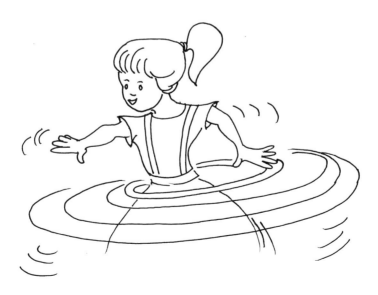

Zoonoses? What Are They, Doc?

Matthew came to me with complaints of a high fever and loose stools. He had been all right a day earlier, running around and breaking things, as three-year-olds do. But that day, just like a clock with a low battery, Matthew slowed down. He complained of severe abdominal cramps, held his tummy with his hands, shivered, and lay down exhausted. Matthew's mother noticed a few streaks of blood in his stool and immediately brought him to my office.

On questioning, Matthew's mother told me that the family hadn't traveled recently, eaten canned or leftover foods, or eaten out. In addition, Matthew hadn't accidentally ingested any medications, and no other family members had diarrhea or were sick.

Matthew's sunken eyes, dry skin, and parched tongue told me that he was severely dehydrated. I immediately admitted him to the hospital. After ordering the proper tests for dehydration and blood and stool cultures, I started him on intravenous fluids and antibiotics. I am glad to say that Matthew improved very fast and was almost back to normal within a couple of days.

The stool culture I sent showed a germ belonging to a group called "salmonella". Having known that these germs sometimes are transmitted from animals to children, I questioned Matthew's mother.

"Do you raise any cattle or pigs?" I asked. The family lived in a rural area.

"No," she replied.

"Chickens or ducks?"

"No."

"Does Matthew have a guinea pig or a hamster?"

"No."

"Pet turtle or snake?"

"Oh, no," she chuckled.

"Well, do you have any pet birds?"

"Yes, we have a few pigeons."

I had the answer I needed.

Salmonella are a type of bacteria that are widely distributed in nature and closely associated with animals. Actually, salmonella were named after the pathologist Salmon who first isolated these germs from a pig's intestine.

Salmonella can infect many creatures, but those hazardous to our health are meat producing animals and poultry. Chickens carrying salmonella infection can contaminate eggs; the germs can penetrate the eggshell and infect the contents. Chickens with infected ovaries can transmit the infection to the egg yolk directly. It is very easy for these germs to enter our kitchens and be transferred to utensils, table surfaces, and to ourselves through contaminated meats and poultry. With poor handwashing, the infection can spread rapidly from person to person.

Ducks, sheep, dogs, cats, turkeys, pigeons, parrots, turtles, and snakes are among the animals whose stools can carry large quantities of salmonella germs, and children playing with these animals can easily get infected if they do not wash properly. It is interesting that rattlesnake meat is used in folk medicine and has caused outbreaks of salmonella infection.

Other food products like bakers' yeast, dried milk, dried

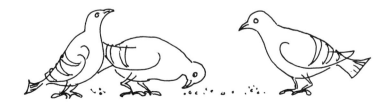

coconut, cottonseed protein, and various dyes can also get contaminated with this germ. Contaminated marijuana has caused this infection as well.

I think that Matthew probably got his salmonella infection through not washing his hands properly after playing with the family pigeons. No other source was found when a public health official inspected the house.

Diseases that are transmitted from animals to humans are called "Zoonoses". When you seek medical help, your doctor may sometimes arrive at a diagnosis sooner if you mention the animals you or your children come into contact with!

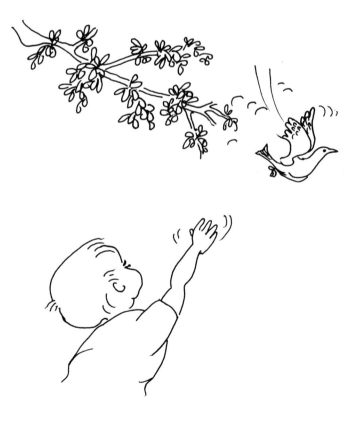

Medical Detectives

*D*octors are like detectives because they investigate and probe into minute details of medical history and lab values to spot a disease. Sometimes a simple question will help to recognize or exclude a disease. Dr. Forman, one of my surgical colleagues, once called me and asked, "Dr. Rao, I have a six-year-old boy, Robert, on the operating table for a ruptured appendix, and I need to operate right now. The lab just told me that Robert has high blood sugar. The lab technician said that the blood was drawn before starting any intravenous (IV) fluids. Robert is probably a diabetic, so how much insulin do you want me to give him? Will you help me?"

Intravenous fluids alter laboratory values, hence blood is usually drawn before starting IV fluids or medications. Newly diagnosed diabetes mellitus needs to be very carefully handled, especially at times of stress such as an infection or an operation; insulin may have to be given intravenously, monitoring blood sugars frequently. Before I ordered insulin for Robert, I had to make sure that Robert had diabetes mellitus. I had to decide fast and I was under pressure.

I told Dr. Forman to hold the insulin, suggested IV fluids without glucose, and requested him to go ahead with the operation. I headed for the lab on the third floor to review the blood sugar values. I knew the lab staff, and located Ruth, who had tended to Robert in the emergency room.

"Ruth," I said, "When you drew blood from Robert, was the IV fluid running in?"

"The first time I drew blood, the ER staff were getting ready to start an IV on him," she said. "The second time I drew blood, he was already getting the fluids."

"That's interesting! Why did you draw it for the second time?"

"Blood in one of the test tubes got spoiled, so I needed to draw another specimen to test for sugar and electrolytes," Ruth explained.

By that time, Robert had received IV fluids with glucose and electrolytes, which probably made his blood sugar go up. Aside from Ruth, nobody else knew about the IV fluids, so when Dr. Forman called, another lab technician mistakenly told him the blood had been drawn before the IV fluids were given.

I told Dr. Forman what had happened. After the operation was over, we repeated a blood sugar test and it was normal; Robert was not a diabetic. His parents were very happy and thanked me for making a correct diagnosis.

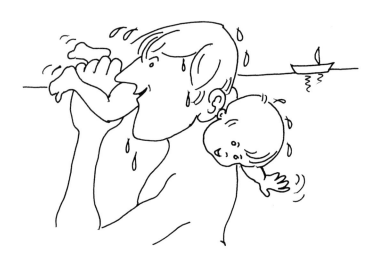

A Singular Case of Seeing Double

*S*ometimes life's very complex problems have simple answers. Such events teach me humility. Take the case of Veronica Gonzalez, four years old, who came to me with complaints of a cold and severe headaches of two weeks duration. Veronica's parents didn't speak English and Veronica only knew a few words. Through an interpreter I learned that several months earlier Veronica had fallen and hit her head. She didn't lose consciousness at that time nor did she have giddiness, weakness, or vomiting. Her parents told me that occasionally she saw things in double.

A thorough examination showed that most things were normal. While checking the nervous system, I stood at the other end of the room and instructed Veronica to count my fingers. I held up one finger and asked, "How many?"

"Two," she replied.

I held three fingers up and asked, "How many?"

"Six."

I showed her two fingers and asked, "How many now?"

"Four," said Veronica.

That was serious. Double vision and headaches following a head injury could mean a blood clot pressing over her brain, or a brain tumor. And there could be many other causes. I made Veronica an appointment with an eye doctor to check for refraction errors. Also, I consulted a neurologist who recommended a CAT scan, appropriate in such a situation. Depending on the scan report, I would refer Veronica to a neurosurgeon if it was a blood clot or to an oncologist if it was a brain tumor. Through an interpreter I explained all this to Veronica's very worried parents.

Veronica's CAT scan showed no tumor or blood clot, but showed evidence of a sinus infection in the frontal bone of the skull. So I gave her an antibiotic. When I saw her ten days later, her headache was gone and she was fit as a fiddle. Could her double vision have gone as well? I held up one finger and asked, "How many?"

Once again she said, "Two."

I held up two fingers and asked, "How many?"

"Five."

I showed her three fingers and asked, "How many?"

"Four."

The truth suddenly dawned on me. Veronica didn't know how to count. In fact she didn't have "Number one" in her vocabulary. Her counting numbers started from two. At home she would identify a pencil as two, which prompted her parents to think that she was seeing double. During her first office visit, it was by mere chance she picked numbers that were double the ones that I tested. Skill in counting numbers develops later than language.

So it turned out that Veronica's headache was due to a sinus infection and her double vision was due to her inability to count, and also to a statistical coincidence. By the way, Veronica knows how to count now.

Simple answers sometimes suffice for a complex problem. Sherlock Holmes would have chuckled and said, "Elementary, Dr. Watson!"

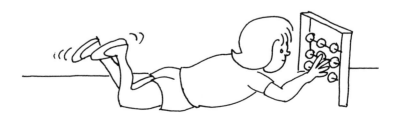

Sphere-Shaped Red Cell Disease

*A*nna, an attractive ten-year-old, came to my office complaining of vomiting, stomach cramps, fatigue, and poor appetite. I discovered that her eyes and skin were yellow, a condition called jaundice. Her liver was palpable, almost an inch below the rib cage margin. These signs and symptoms pointed to an infection of the liver called hepatitis. I requested several tests that measured her liver functions and identified the type of hepatitis.

The test results showed an increase in liver enzymes. Tests for hepatitis A, B, and C were negative. Bilirubin, a yellow pigment that is excreted by the liver in the bile, was elevated in Anna's blood; this was the reason for her yellow colored skin and eyes.

Bilirubin is a very interesting pigment. There are two kinds of bilirubins, indirect and direct. When red blood cells (RBC) get destroyed in large numbers, a condition that is called hemolysis, increased amounts of bilirubin are produced as a byproduct. The liver cannot excrete the excessive amounts of bilirubin efficiently; the bilirubin then backs up and accumulates in the blood, causing jaundice. This bilirubin, the byproduct of red cell destruction, is more water-soluble, and is called indirect bilirubin.

In another scenario, bile is stored in the gallbladder and is emptied into the intestines through a tube called the bile duct. When the duct is obstructed, as with a gallstone blocking the tube, bilirubin backs up in the blood and causes jaundice. This bilirubin is less soluble and is called direct bilirubin. In other words, the presence of elevated indirect bilirubin indicates hemolysis, and increased direct bilirubin points to obstruction of the bile flow.

Anna had elevated indirect and direct bilirubins. I requested several tests to diagnose hemolysis and obstruction to bile flow. During one of the visits, Anna's mother casually asked me, "Dr. Rao, I have spherocytosis. Do you think Anna's problems are also due to this condition?"

That was it! I went to the lab and examined Anna's blood smear. While normal red cells are biconcave discs with a clear center, Anna's red cells were smaller than normal without the central pallor; in fact, the red cells were like tiny spheres. Anna, like her mother, had a disease known as spherocytosis.

Spherocytosis is an inherited disorder that affects 1 in 5,000 children. Anna's mother, grandmother, and probably her great-grandmother had the disease as well. In this disease, the red cell membrane is defective and hence the cells assume the shape of small spheres called spherocytes. These spherocytes cannot pass through the spaces in the spleen, which is an organ lying in the left upper part of the abdomen. The spherocytes stagnate in the spleen and are destroyed, producing increased amounts of bilirubin and causing jaundice. Prolonged, excessive bile pigment excretion through the gallbladder produces gallstones. Anna's abdominal sonogram showed gallstones; that is how Anna had elevated direct and indirect bilirubins in her blood.

Anna was referred to a nearby hospital. There, her spleen was removed to prevent further destruction of her red cells. She was also put on prophylactic antibiotics. Anna looked more lively and active the last time I saw her, but she will have those sphere-shaped red cells throughout her life.

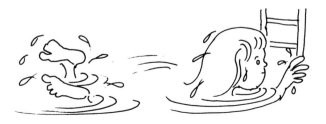

Doctor Dog, Ace Cancer Spotter

*D*ogs rescue stranded skiers, save people from drowning, guide the blind, sniff out drugs and bombs, and aid in investigations of arson. What is less well known is that children with chronic diseases and disabilities recover sooner when in company with a dog. Dogs help people with Parkinson's disease, making their lives more comfortable by doing simple chores like turning the lights on and off, picking fallen objects, and preventing falls. Some dogs can sense seizures 30 minutes before they occur, and warn their masters, who then will lie down, avoiding injuries. Now, are you ready to believe that man's best friend can diagnose diseases too?

A 44-year-old woman had multiple moles over her body. Her dog, half Border Collie, half Doberman, kept sniffing repeatedly at a mole over her thigh, and once tried to bite it off. The woman was concerned and consulted a doctor; the mole on her thigh was removed and later proved to be a melanoma, a bad cancer of the skin. The dog had literally saved the woman's life, and the episode was duly recorded in the medical journal, *Lancet*, in 1959.

Dr. Armand Cognetta, a dermatologist in Tallahassee, noticed the report. As a dog's sense of smell is 300 times more sensitive than a human's, Dr. Cognetta felt he could train a dog to sniff and diagnose melanoma. With help from Duane Pickel, a veteran dog trainer, he managed to train a schnauzer called George to identify the cancer. First, George was trained to find, among numerous test tubes, the only one that contained melanoma cells. Then he was trained to find the melanoma sample when it was hidden in one of many holes in a box. George was able to sniff out the correct one with remarkable accuracy. Next, the researchers hid the cancer cells in a bandage on a person who was covered with many bandages. George could sniff the cancer 100 percent of the time. Then George was trained to examine a patient with multiple moles or suspected melanoma.

How did George examine a patient? Dr. Cognetta and Mr. Pickel designed an examination table that stood close to the ground. When a patient lay down, George was given a command, and he would then sniff the patient from head to toe. If melanoma was present, George would place his paw over the area where he smelled the cancer. George was correct 99 percent of the time.

As dogs' noses are far more sensitive than those of humans, dogs are now being trained to detect several diseases that have characteristic odors. For example, surgeons at Cambridge University plan to test the dog's capability to detect cancers of the prostate by sniffing patient's urine.

Having a dog sniff you to find out whether you have melanoma is interesting, but not an ideal way of finding the disease. Consider taking preventive measures instead, by using sunscreen and checking skin moles regularly for changes in size, shape, color, and bleeding. And please see your doctor regularly.

HMOs are increasingly questioning physicians about the need for sophisticated diagnostic tests like CT scans and MRIs. To avoid hassles, I think I will get me a disease-sniffing dog for my office!

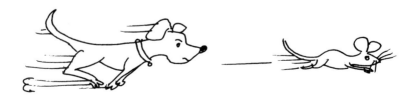

When a "Wrong" Blood Group Can Be Right

I have known Mr. and Mrs. Land for a long time; they are a very nice family and have brought their children to my office for several years. I was therefore happy when Mrs. Land brought her newborn infant, Lisa, in for a check-up.

Lisa was healthy. As Mrs. Land was dressing Lisa to leave, she hesitated, "Dr. Rao, my husband is telling me to check Lisa's blood group. The problem is this. My blood group is A and my husband's is B. In the newborn nursery they told us that Lisa's blood group is O. How can that be? My husband says Lisa's group should be A or B or AB. There must be an error somewhere. Can you please give me a lab slip to check Lisa's blood group again?"

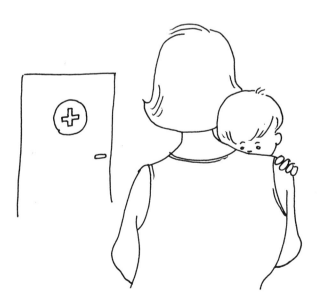

I was very concerned, as I knew well the implications involved in such requests. Having had a similar experience when I was a fellow in hematology, I was careful not to make any comment, but excused myself and grabbed a hematology textbook. Using the textbook as a reference, I charted the four common blood groups of imaginary parents and possible blood groups that their children could inherit. The chart looked like this:

Parents' Blood		Possible Blood Groups Groups In Their Children
A	A	A, O
B	B	B, O
A	B	A, B, AB, O
A	AB	A, B, AB
A	O	A, O
B	AB	A, B, AB
B	O	B, O
AB	AB	A, B, AB
AB	O	A, B
O	O	O

"Mrs. Land, you can see on line three that parents of A and B blood groups can have a child with an O blood group," I pointed out.

"How did the O group come from A and B group parents?" was her next question.

A little more explanation was needed. Even though Mrs. Land had the A blood group, her genetic makeup, called the genotype, was very likely AO. She inherited each of these components from her parents. In her husband with the B group, the genetic makeup was likely BO. Their children would have the following genetic make-ups (genotypes), namely, AB, AO, OO, and BO. These correspond to actual blood groups AB, A, O, and B respectively. Every time the Lands had a child, their child had a one-in-four chance of inheriting any one of the blood groups mentioned above. It so happened that Lisa inherited the O blood group. Blood groups and their genotypes are noted below.

Blood Group	Genotypes
O	OO
A	AA, AO
B	BB, BO
AB	AB

I briefly explained the inheritance pattern to Mrs. Land, and she left my office very happy.

In 1940 Charlie Chaplin was involved in a paternity case. His blood group was O, the child's group was B, and the mother's blood group was A. Using the data given in my story, can you tell if Chaplin was the father of the child?

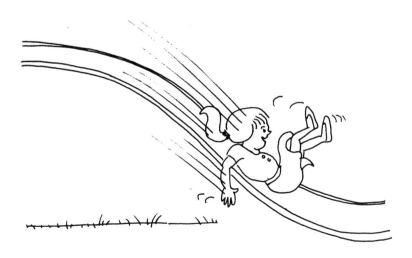

Can This Syndrome Make You Lie?

"Doctor, how old do you think the bruise was when you examined Mary's foot?" asked the defense lawyer, when I had taken the stand. "It was pink in color and looked fresh. I would say that it was less than 12 hours old," I replied.

"Did you see any shoe marks on Mary's foot?"

"No, I saw a few scratch marks."

"Doctor, please answer yes or no. Were there any shoe marks on her foot?"

"No."

"Medical records show that Mary had slipped and fallen over the footpath a day before. Is it possible that she could have sustained the bruise then?"

"Yes, it's possible."

"Have you reviewed Mary's records recently?" asked the attorney.

"Yes."

"To the best of your knowledge, what disease does Mary have?"

"Prader-Willi Syndrome."

"Is it not true, the attorney continued, "that patients affected with this disease have developmental delays and behavioral problems?"

"Yes."

"Then, is it possible that Mary could have falsely accused my client of having stepped on her foot?"

"Yes, it's possible."

"That's all, your Honor." The defense attorney sat down with a smile.

The prosecution attorney asked, "Doctor, can the scratch marks on Mary's foot be caused by a shoe rubbing on her foot without leaving a shoe print?"

"Yes."

"Do people with Prader-Willi Syndrome always lie?"

"No," I replied.

"Because her foot was stamped upon and it hurt, is it possible that Mary was telling the truth this time?"

"That is possible."

"That's all, your honor."

Mary had complained that her caretaker had stepped on her foot intentionally. Someone had seen the incident and reported it to the proper authorities. As the accused contested the charge, the case came to court.

Mary had a disease called Prader-Willi Syndrome. Prader described it in 1956; it occurs about once in 25,000 births. The disease is due to a deletion of a small segment of chromosome 15; interestingly, in this disease the chromosome 15 that is affected is always paternally derived.

Babies born with this disease have severe muscle weakness. They suck poorly and some need to be tube fed. Interestingly, this muscle weakness improves by 8 to 11 months. By the age of one to two years, however, these children develop delayed psychomotor impairment and increased appetite. They consume large quantities of food and gain enormous amounts of weight. They appear short with small hands and feet and have almond shaped eyes. As they grow, they develop endocrine problems such as diabetes, breathing difficulties, cardiovascular problems, abnormal behaviors, and retardation.

There is no cure for the disease. Controlling the weight by strict dieting, attending to cardiovascular and lung problems, and giving support as needed is all that can be done. Patients can lead a normal life, but some are institutionalized when their retardation is severe.

I attended to Mary's bruise. X rays of her foot were normal and her bruise healed in a few days.

One has to be very careful in assessing accusations by mentally retarded or delayed persons. In such instances, circumstantial evidence can help to uncover the truth. Later I came to know that the accused was found not guilty.

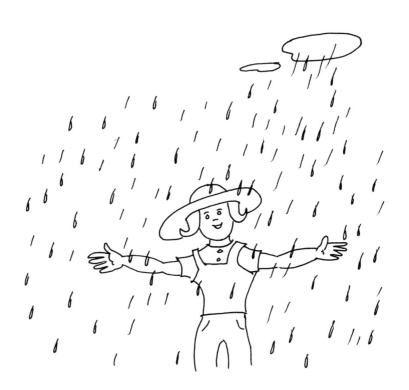

An Odd Cause for Vomiting Blood

Mrs. Cox brought Destiny, her cute six-month-old infant, to my office with a history of vomiting blood, a condition called hematemesis. Mrs. Cox told me that Destiny threw up milk mixed with blood twice in the past two days. Initially she had thought that Destiny had vomited juice, but when it happened the second time, she got scared and brought Destiny to my office.

Through an interpreter, I asked Mrs. Cox about a family history of bleeding disorders; there was none. Destiny had not been given any aspirin, which could have irritated the stomach and caused hematemesis. There was no history of any ingestion of toxic chemicals or sharp objects, neither was there any injury to the abdomen. Destiny hadn't had a nosebleed that would have caused her to swallow blood and vomit it later.

As I examined Destiny, I noticed a slight redness of her gums due to teething; however, there was no bleeding from the gums. The throat was not congested and there were no bruises or pinpoint bleeding spots, called petechiae, on the skin. Her lymph glands were normal, and her spleen and liver were not enlarged. All these indicated an absence of any obvious cause for Destiny's hematemesis.

Hematemesis in six-month-olds can be due to a variety of conditions such as inflammation of the foodpipe or stomach, ulcers, foreign bodies, dilated blood vessels called varices, and aneurysms. If it was a blood vessel malformation, what made it bleed at six months? Allergy to formulas containing cow's milk usually causes microscopic bleeding, not copious hematemesis.

"What kind of formula are you feeding Destiny?" I asked Mrs. Cox.

"I'm still breast-feeding the baby. It hurts when she nurses," she replied.

After further questioning, Mrs. Cox confided that there were small fissures around the site of nursing, which bled minimally. Mrs.Cox did not think much of it, but when Destiny nursed vigorously, she swallowed small quantities of blood from the fissures, and because the blood probably irritated her stomach, she vomited. That was how blood came into Destiny's vomitus.

I advised Mrs. Cox to call her own doctor to treat the fissures, and told her to stop nursing the baby until the lesions healed. Destiny stopped vomiting blood and tests for blood in her stools became negative.

I learned something, too—an unusual cause for hematemesis, which books don't usually mention. Children do teach us, if we care to learn!

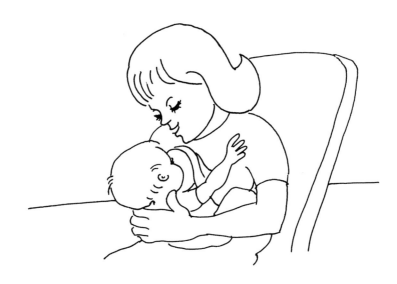

Mystery of the Missing Cells—
Anemia in a Newborn

$\mathcal{S}$ haron was born by cesarean section, weighed about six pounds, and cried vigorously at birth. Physically I did not find anything wrong with her. However, a routine blood count at birth showed a hemoglobin level of 7.5 g/dl, indicating severe anemia. Normal values at birth range between 14.5 and 22.5 g/dl. Other components of her blood, like white cells and platelets, were normal. Her reticulocytes, which are red cells younger than four days, were low, indicating that her bone marrow was not producing red cells effectively. Sharon was in big trouble.

I transferred Sharon to a nearby hospital. She received packed red cell transfusions that raised her hemoglobin to 11.4 g/dl; she did well and was sent home.

Many factors can cause anemia in newborns. We ruled out blood group incompatibility by checking the blood groups, and by conducting a special test called Coombs' test. Sometimes, while still in the womb, babies may bleed into their mother's circulation and thus become anemic. This too was ruled out by looking for fetal cells in the mothers' circulation. In yet other newborns, viral infections cause a temporary shutdown of marrow, causing anemia. This was my hope and I expected Sharon to recover within a short time.

Unexpectedly, Sharon was brought to the emergency room at the age of three months. She did not suck well and she was pale. Her blood counts showed very severe anemia, with a hemoglobin that had dropped to 1.7 g/dl. Once again her white cell and platelet counts were normal, but somehow she was not producing red blood cells. Her blood was so thin and so inefficient in carrying oxygen, that her heart was beating very fast to increase the circulation. Sharon was going into heart failure.

This was very serious. I transferred her to a nearby children's hospital, brooding over the rare blood diseases that could be affecting Sharon.

A bone marrow aspiration on Sharon showed a complete absence of red cell precursors, though her white cell and platelet precursors were normal. These findings confirmed my suspicion that Sharon had a rare disorder called "Diamond-Blackfan Syndrome" or "congenital hypoplastic anemia". So far only a very few children have been described as having this disorder.

Sharon received packed red cell transfusions. She was also started on prednisone because three-fourths of children with Diamond-Blackfan Syndrome respond favorably to it. Sharon needed several transfusions that year. Later she started to produce red cells on prednisone and maintained her hemoglobin around 8 g/dl. Indeed it is a wonder drug!

The last I saw Sharon, she was on a very low dose of prednisone, given on alternate days. Her growth in height was impaired, probably due to the prednisone therapy. However, a few children with this disorder are short-statured. Sharon had osteoporosis that improved after the prednisone dosage was cut.

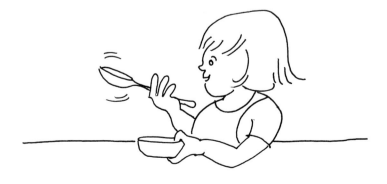

The Joy of Small Things

Ritchie was born to a 16-year-old mother during Halloween, and had severe birth injury during delivery. Either due to that or to some other unknown cause, he developed mental retardation. When Ritchie's mother was 18, she got divorced and could not take care of him. As everyone predicted, there was no hope of improvement for Ritchie, and he was placed in a home. There, many Halloweens came and went.

Ritchie developed severe spasticity of his extremities; that is to say, he had limited movement of his arms and legs. He did not have self-help skills, yet, in spite of several handicaps, over the years he had patiently mastered a few simple tasks.

I used to stand at the glass door of the corridor that led to his room. Ritchie would look at me with his myopic eyes and laugh; more a grunt than a laugh, it was a sign of recognition. Then he would push and maneuver his wheelchair with his toes—that was the only way he could move—and approach a switch, the size of a small pizza plate. Since he had very limited movement of his arms, he would push the switch with his forehead to open the automatic door to let me in.

My "thanks" would make him laugh in grunts. The door would close automatically and Ritchie would wait patiently behind the door, ready to open it if someone else showed up or his foster grandparent came to take him out.

Ritchie liked to paint but could not, as he could not hold a brush with his spastic fingers. The wonderful occupational therapist at that home custom-made him a universal cuff that could hold a long brush in place. With limited movements at the elbow and wrist, Ritchie managed to dip the brush in the paint and scribble on the canvas, producing simple designs. Later, he would grunt and demand that the paintings be hung in the hallway. He would eye them and laugh with happiness.

Ritchie loved bowling as a leisure activity. His caretakers had a special bowling rack for handicapped people. Since Ritchie could not use his hands, but was adept at using his head, the therapist made him a special helmet to wear during bowling. Ritchie would push the ball with his special helmet and watch it roll. At such times his joy knew no bounds.

For his daily classes Ritchie had to make a trip up a wheel-chair ramp. He would patiently push the wheelchair backward with his right foot, inch by inch, until he reached the ramp's upper end. This would take almost ten minutes. Sometimes, exhausted, he would stop and tumble in his wheelchair down the ramp, where his ever-vigilant caretakers would catch him. Other residents waiting at the lower end would laugh at this fiasco.

In our rat-race lives, we fail to take time to notice simple things around us. Just like an asthmatic can truly appreciate the joy of normal breathing, Ritchie helped me notice the joy in simple acts like pushing a wheelchair or opening the door with his fore-head. He taught me that the greatest happiness sometimes lies in simple acts.

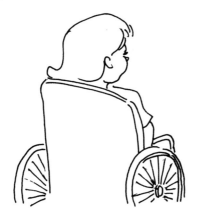
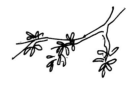

A Winning Bout with Leukemia

*T*he very first snapshot of Danny I have in my memory is that of a newborn. Danny's mother brought him to my office for a sore throat, which I treated with an antibiotic. Danny was a cute little boy with plenty of black hair. I remember him kicking vigorously as I checked him that day.

I remember Danny next as a toddler who came to my office with a history of nosebleeds and blisters in his mouth. Apart from a sore throat, I found petechiae—pinpoint-sized bleeding spots—over his skin. Blood tests revealed that he had a low platelet count and an abnormal increase in lymphocytes.

Platelets, one of the components of blood, are essential for clotting. When they are low, bleeding occurs. Lymphocytes are a part of our body's defense system, and typically increase in viral infections. However, a combination of low platelets and increased lymphocytes usually implies a serious problem. Hence, I examined Danny's blood smear. My suspicion proved to be correct: Danny had leukemia. I sent him to a children's hospital for treatment.

The next snapshot is when Danny walked into my office at 22 months of age. He had a Broviac catheter stuck onto his chest wall so strong medications could go directly into a blood vessel. His skin was peculiar. There were dark patches with some small areas of vitiligo-like lesions; that is to say, white discoloration appeared on parts of his body. Also, some areas of his skin were peeling off. What was happening to Danny?

The children's hospital had diagnosed acute myelogenous leukemia, and after initial treatment had sent Danny to a university hospital where he was to receive his elder brother's bone marrow.

There, Danny then received medications and radiation prior to the marrow transplant to kill the leukemic cells and suppress his own immune system. After the transplant, however, a fresh complication arose: the transplanted cells began to produce antibodies against Danny's body cells. So, it was not Danny's cells that were rejecting the transplanted cells, but his brother's cells that were rejecting Danny's cells. This kind of reaction is called "graft versus host disease". That was why Danny's skin cells were peeling off. What a situation!

Danny was given medications to counteract the graft versus host disease. The treatment had to be carefully monitored: too strong and too high doses would cause the sibling's transplanted cells to shut off. If, on the other hand, the doses were too small, Danny's own cells would be rejected. The medicines were carefully adjusted and a delicate balance was obtained. It turned into a constant but bearable fight between Danny's cells and his brother's cells.

The last snapshot is of Danny at 18. Due to the medications and graft versus host disease, Danny is a little short for his age and weighs only 85 pounds, but there is no evidence of leukemia. He is in the 12th grade and has plans to go to college.

Life is an album of snapshots of events and experiences. Some are good, some are not good. I like Danny's album, though, because the last snapshot is just right!

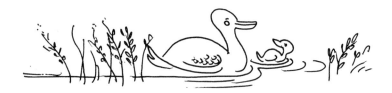

Living Moment to Moment

"Hi, grandpa!" Peter said. Although he was a teenager, he lived in a nursing home. He pulled around a toy wagon with a basketball inside, and greeted everyone he met as "grandpa" or "rat" or any other whimsical name he concocted.

If you had seen Peter walking around nonchalantly, dragging his wagon and basketball, you would never have guessed the multiple medical problems he suffered from. In addition to seizures and a thyroid problem, Peter had kidney failure. He received seizure and thyroid medications, and dialysis to alleviate his problems. Though he also had temper tantrums and was developmentally disabled, those handicaps did not prevent him from taking part in his daily activities.

Peter knew how to dress himself and use the toilet. He disliked making his bed and sought help from caretakers. He ate his food with a spoon. After breakfast or lunch, he would locate his toy wagon and place an empty box or a ball inside the wagon. This was done ritualistically, and he would drag the wagon around the nursing home and greet people here and there. He would stop by at a nursing station, ask for a cup of coffee and sit there chatting with people. Sometimes he would sit on a bench under a tree, seemingly enjoying these moments while sipping his coffee.

Evenings, after dinner, Peter showered and watched movies. If it was a cowboy movie, it made his day. At such times he socialized with peers and caretakers, and this is how a typical day ended for him.

One day I was walking by, when I saw Peter as he sat on a

bench beneath a tree, sipping coffee. His pet wagon with a ball was nearby, and he was very happy.

"Peter," I said, "why are you so happy?"

"I don't know," he replied. Then he added, "Coffee."

Simple things like coffee, dragging a toy wagon, or watching a cowboy movie made Peter very happy. It seemed to me then that the rest of us are either stranded in past memories or worry too much about the unborn future. We should learn to live in the present, moment by moment, enjoying the simple things in life, as Peter did in spite of all his handicaps.

On my way back, there was Peter again. "Hi, grandpa," he said.

"Not a grandpa yet," I replied, before moving on with a much lighter step, thinking about my newly wed daughter living far away.

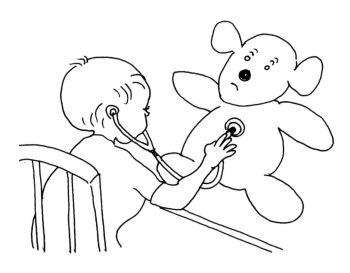

A Very Brave Girl's Battle With Muscular Atrophy

I have known Patricia almost since her birth; I remember her cute face and abundant hair. When Mrs. Pankhurst, Patricia's mother, first came to my office, she filled out a questionnaire indicating a healthy family history. Except for iron deficiency anemia at the age of 18 months, which I treated with iron, Patricia's infancy was unremarkable.

At four years of age Patricia walked with her toes turned inwards like a pigeon, and had difficulty running. I examined her thoroughly and found a mild weakness at her ankle joints. She also had a foot-drop. Her intelligence was normal.

Many diseases cause these signs and symptoms. I scratched my head trying to chart a course to diagnose Patricia's condition quickly and easily.

At that juncture Mrs. Pankhurst told me an interesting family history. She too had had foot drop, in-toeing, and difficulty walking when she was young. She needed several corrective operations on her legs and wore braces, but walks well now. Patricia's maternal grandmother also had this problem and still walked. Patricia's aunt and a cousin had similar problems. Even though Mrs. Pankhurst forgot the name of the disease, it was easy to figure it out—Patricia had a hereditary disease called "Charcot-Marie-Tooth Disease". A neurologist later confirmed the diagnosis and I arranged for genetic counseling and orthopedic evaluations.

Charcot-Marie-Tooth disease has nothing to do with tooth disorders. Doctors Martin Charcot, Pierre Marie, and Howard

Tooth described this condition in 1886 and hence the name. This disease is also called "Peroneal Muscular Atrophy", as the peroneal muscles located in the legs get atrophied. It is a disorder inherited as a dominant trait; this means that a parent with the defective gene can transmit the disease and there is a 50 percent chance that a child will get it. Children of either sex are equally affected. The incidence is 1 in 26,315.

Children with Charcot-Marie-Tooth Disease show progressive muscle weakness in their feet, lower legs, hands, and forearms. They may develop a loss of sensation in the areas mentioned, but longevity and intelligence are not affected. Most patients walk, although orthotic appliances are needed to stabilize the ankles.

The last time I saw Patricia, she was undergoing physical therapy and was able to walk with braces. She was in the seventh grade. She had seen her grandmother, mother, aunt, and a cousin struggle through this handicap. As she walked slowly out of my office she knew exactly what lay ahead and was prepared to meet the challenge of her life with a smile. Life shrinks or expands in proportion to one's courage. Patricia was a very brave girl!

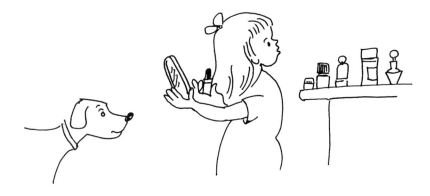

She Won Against Cancer

I saw Brenda, a fifteen-year-old Mexican girl, for nodules in her neck. Brenda's pediatrician had treated her with antibiotics for tonsillitis and enlarged glands. As the size of the glands remained the same, Brenda's pediatrician requested me to evaluate her.

Brenda had huge lymph glands on both sides of her neck, and slightly enlarged glands just above her collarbones, in her armpits, and groin area. They were not painful. Her throat infection was gone. Otherwise she looked healthy. After a few preliminary blood tests, Brenda underwent a lymph gland biopsy, which showed a type of cancer called lymphoblastic lymphoma. Furthermore, a bone marrow biopsy showed cancer cells, and a CAT scan of the abdomen revealed enlarged lymph glands along the major blood vessels. This was bad news. Brenda's cancer had spread all over her body.

In the short period of a week, Brenda's dreams of graduating from school, going in for higher education, dating, getting married, and raising a family were shattered. Instead, she faced radiation treatments, week after week of chemotherapy, innumerable blood drawings, and bone marrow aspirations. Moreover, nobody was sure whether she would be cured. Statistics about patients who were free of the disease after treatment did not make any sense to Brenda. She was depressed.

But Brenda had assets that many don't have. She had a very positive attitude about life and a good relationship with her family. Her parents were emotionally stable, religiously oriented and had satisfying jobs. They supported Brenda to the hilt, day and night with unconditional love; in turn they got support from an extended family of brothers and sisters.

"Why me?" Brenda asked me one day.

"That's a very difficult question to answer," I told her. "Certain chemicals, radiation, and chromosomal abnormalities are known to cause cancer. You were not exposed to chemicals or radiation, and we didn't find any chromosomal defects in you. One day, science will advance so much that we will be able to tell why a person gets cancer, but we are not there yet."

Brenda's mother had another explanation. "God tests good people by challenging them with tough problems," she said. "He wants to know whether you can stand up to the challenge."

"How long do I need to take these poisons?" Brenda asked.

"For about a year and a half," I replied. "Nowadays there is a 70 percent chance of being disease-free after chemotherapy."

Brenda ignored my statistics.

"Will I lose hair?"

"Yes, but when we stop chemotherapy, you will grow it back. Meanwhile you may wear a wig. My professor once had told me that an African American child she treated later grew hair without kinks."

Brenda laughed.

After a short course of radiation treatment to her neck glands, which melted away like butter, Brenda was started on a long course of chemotherapy. To facilitate that, a catheter was put into one of her chest veins.

As the chemotherapy progressed, Brenda's hair fell off, just a few strands in the beginning, and then in clumps. The medical center gave her a wig. Brenda wore it a couple of days, hating it, and finally threw it out. She did not want to attend the school bald. By and by, she mustered enough courage and went to school. A handful of students made fun of her, but the majority rallied to her side and criticized the insensitive classmates. Her friends' support made Brenda realize that people cared for her, and friendship and love were more important than appearances.

Brenda's parents stood by her day and night. When there was a party, they took her along even though she could stay only for a few minutes. While Brenda was in bed, they encouraged her to do small tasks—to rearrange the sheets a little, or dust off the side table, just to keep her occupied and break the monotony.

There were times when, late at night, Brenda was sleepless, and would cry and ask her mother whether she would make it. Her mother would reply in a soothing voice, "My child, I don't have any doubts that you will make it. You will, you will." At other times she would reply, "Brenda, you are a child. You haven't had time to sin yet. So I'm sure that if the unthinkable happens, you'll go to heaven. For me, I'm not sure, as I have lived longer and hence might have sinned without my knowledge. I'm getting older and you have the responsibility to take care of your sister, Jodi. Being defeated is usually a temporary condition. Giving up is what makes it permanent. You have a purpose in life so don't give up easily. I love you." Brenda would hug her mother and the long nights would pass as her silent tears soaked the pillow.

Finally, after a year and a half, we stopped the chemotherapy. Brenda was happy that it was over. I was happy there was no evidence of cancer.

Brenda picked up the loose ends of her life and completed the required courses in school. She received her high school diploma and enrolled in our local community college. Her cheerfulness and zest for life returned.

At about that time, Brenda began to feel pain in her hips and began limping. I ordered X rays and a CAT scan, which showed degenerative changes in her hip joints. This could have been an effect of chemotherapy or infiltration of cancer cells in her hip joints. The only way to know was to get a piece of hip tissue by operation and study it under a microscope.

Brenda was devastated but her family rallied to her side. Didn't Brenda win the first round against the cancer devil with

God's help? She would do it again. She should have faith in Him and pray; He would take all the pain and suffering for her. She would be well again. She should keep moving. Life is like riding a bicycle. One didn't fall off unless one stopped pedaling.

The biopsy showed no evidence of cancer, but confirmed that there were degenerative changes, probably due to chemotherapy. Brenda was relieved. She just needed crutches and painkillers.

Once again, Brenda picked up the pieces and strove to make a sensible picture of her life. Gradually recovering her self-confidence, she studied hard in spite of her nagging hip pain and limp. It took a little longer, but she graduated from college.

Then Brenda fell in love. This raised concerns: cancer treatment often impacts late on childbearing organs. Ovaries may get damaged and not produce eggs; adhesions may develop in the tubes. All these prevent conception. On the other hand, many successful pregnancies have occurred and healthy infants have been born to mothers who underwent cancer therapy. In Brenda's case, however, she might not be able to carry a pregnancy to term because of her hip problems.

Her doctor expressed these concerns, but Brenda had different ideas. She felt that she needed to enjoy life to the fullest. She wanted to have a child. She told her mother, "I took a chance with my life in combating cancer. Mom, I will take another chance in having a child. Who knows? I may win. If not, I still will have the satisfaction that I tried."

Brenda had a healthy baby girl; the last I knew, she was a year-and-a-half old and a bundle of joy to her mother. For her part, Brenda was learning medical accounting and hoped to get a job in the medical field.

I believe Brenda's success was due to her strong willpower, her belief in herself, her faith in God, and the unflinching support she received from family and friends. Despite innumerable problems, Brenda came through with flying colors.

It Takes a Village

One day Mrs. Duran asked me whether I would examine Pedro, her nephew, who had muscle weakness. Mrs. Duran told me that one of Pedro's maternal uncles had had muscle weakness and had died. I agreed to check Pedro, but I did not realize how far she needed to go to bring him to my office. He lived in a small village in Mexico.

Pedro was a cheerful six-year-old. I examined him thoroughly. He walked peculiarly, with a waddle like a duck. When I asked him to get up from a sitting position on the floor, he did so by pushing his body up with his hands against the ankles, knees, and thighs. This was due to a weakness in his hip muscles. Using the hands to "climb up" the legs in order to assume an upright posture is called "Gowers sign". The rest of his examination was normal.

In some muscle diseases, an enzyme called "creatinine kinase" is increased, indicating muscle degeneration. In Pedro, this enzyme was enormously elevated. His family history, his muscle weakness, and the enzyme elevation all pointed to a sinister disease known as "Duchenne Muscular Dystrophy". After consulting experts, a muscle biopsy confirmed the diagnosis.

Duchenne muscular dystrophy is inherited through the sex chromosome "X" in a recessive manner. Females carry the disease and usually have no symptoms, but pass it on to male children, who develop the illness.

The disease progresses relentlessly. Hip muscles are affected first, followed by the shoulder muscles. Children with the disease get progressively weaker, and need a wheelchair by the age of ten. Slowly, they develop flexion contractures of the arms and legs, as well as spinal deformities. The heart muscle also gets affected. Throat muscles become weak, leading to aspiration of food. As the years go by, the respiratory muscles become weak and breathing becomes difficult. Finally, these children die at about the age of 18, due to aspirations, lung infections, respiratory failure, or heart problems. What a terrible disease to inherit!

Although at the time of writing several experimental treatments are being attempted, including gene therapy, there is still neither a cure nor a way to stop the relentless progress of this disease. Physiotherapy and good nutrition were all that we could offer Pedro. Mrs. Duran was sad to hear the outcome of Pedro's illness, yet she was satisfied that we were able to make a definitive diagnosis and explain the inheritance pattern. With a heavy heart I bade Pedro goodbye as he left my office to go back to his village in Mexico.

I kept getting news about Pedro through Mrs. Duran for a couple of years. By and by he became weaker and could not walk, but his family and friends in the village solved his ambulatory problem in a unique way—they bought him a pony. Since his upper body was still strong, he could control the pony; he felt very happy and loved it and the unexpected freedom it brought into his life. For their part, his family and friends were happy that they could help Pedro in the declining days of his life. Those who bring sunshine to the lives of others cannot keep it from themselves.

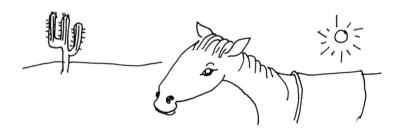

Unsung Heroes of Society

$\mathcal{A}$ndrea came into the world blue and limp. Immediately, she was intubated and given oxygen. When she was stable, X rays showed an abnormal elevation of her diaphragm over the right side. The diaphragm is a muscle that separates the chest from the abdomen and is essential for breathing; when part of it protrudes into the chest—a condition called eventration—the child cannot breathe properly and becomes blue due to lack of oxygen. If this continues for even a few minutes, damage occurs to the brain, the heart, and to other organs.

Andrea had a stormy course at the hospital. She needed oxygen for six days, digoxin to pep her heart, intravenous fluids, and antibiotics. She slowly recovered, but the lack of oxygen had already damaged her brain, a condition that is called hypoxic encephalopathy. Because of that, she had weak muscles, and poor sucking and swallowing. Her mother was instructed to stimulate Andrea's lips and mouth, which she patiently did so that Andrea could suck better. As there was no improvement, Andrea eventually needed to be fed by a tube. Andrea's mother became very adept at inserting the tube for feeding purposes.

As the weeks passed by, the effects of Andrea's brain damage became apparent. She could not swallow the formula properly, and when solid foods were tried, she choked. Consequently she had very poor weight gain. Investigations showed that Andrea had gastro-esophageal reflux, commonly known as heartburn. Eventually, an operation corrected the reflux; a tube was also introduced into her stomach through the abdominal wall to facilitate feeding. Thus, to some extent, her feeding problem was solved.

As the years passed, Andrea developed dislocation of her hip and scoliosis. In spite of these physical handicaps and mental disability, Andrea slowly learned to speak, first single words, then a few simple sentences with a drawl. Her apprehension in my office slowly vanished, giving way to smiles. Her mother constantly encouraged Andrea to learn. I was happy to see her progress.

One day, while coming out of the examination room, I saw Andrea moving her hand in a peculiar way. By now she was 11 years old.

"What is she doing?" I asked the mother.

"Andrea, show the doctor," her mother prompted her. Andrea slowly made a fist of her left hand and extended her thumb. She smiled gingerly and said, "A". Then ever so slowly she extended her fingers and put her thumb across her palm and said, "B". I realized that Andrea was proudly showing me the alphabet of the sign language she had learned. I was flabbergasted. I was amazed at Andrea's mother, too; day after day, patiently for three years, she had taught her daughter sign language. Because of her persistent efforts, Andrea improved a little by little.

Mothers of children with cerebral palsy or mental retardation, who strive day by day, against all odds, to improve the quality of life for their little ones, are to be commended for their devotion to a noble cause. In my view, they are the real heroes in our society.

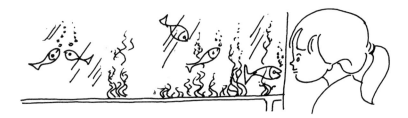

Born Lucky

$\mathcal{M}$eena was born to parents in India who had lost two young children to unknown illnesses. Hence Meena was very precious to them, and when, soon after being born, she began feeding poorly and developed repeated infections, her parents became very worried. When Meena was two months old, her mother traveled to the United States and left Meena with her aunt, Kalyani, for evaluation by experts.

I saw Meena a couple of times while she was being thoroughly investigated in the nearby children's hospital. Specialists in genetics and metabolic diseases had noted that Meena was still feeding poorly and had repeated bouts of fever and diarrhea. She needed antibiotics frequently. In addition, her muscles were weak (hypotonic) and she didn't have much energy.

Meena underwent many tests, and for the most part the results were normal. As disorders of fat metabolism cause similar signs and symptoms, specific tests were carried out that showed elevated levels of dicarboxylic acids in her urine, and low levels of a protein called carnitine in her blood. Meena had a metabolic disorder called "Glutaric Aciduria, Type II".

What are these dicarboxylic acids and carnitine? Why was the former elevated and the latter too low in Meena?

Fat is a good source of energy, but fat in the form of fatty acids has to be broken down to simpler forms by various enzymes with long names, such as "Electron Transfer Flavoprotein Dehydrogenase", "Aceyl Co-enzyme A", and so on. In the absence of these enzymes, fat cannot be broken down completely; several intermediate products like dicarboxylic acids are formed, which accumulate in the cells. Some of these products are very toxic to the cells. Hence, the child develops low blood sugar, vomiting, seizures, and other symptoms.

Many children with glutaric aciduria have carnitine deficiency. Carnitine is a protein that transports fatty acids into the cell mitochondria. When carnitine is low, fatty acids cannot be mobilized and metabolized. This adds fuel to the fire. More intermediate toxic products accumulate, causing further damage to the cells. The child may die if not treated promptly.

Meena was put on a diet restricted in fat. As her carnitine was low, she was started on carnitine by mouth. She improved remarkably and was able to handle infections better. At the age of two years she could speak English in addition to her mother tongue. She went back to India to join her happy parents. The last I heard, Meena was developing normally and doing well, but she will need to take carnitine for a long time.

Many children in developing countries die due to a lack of expertise in handling this complex disorder. Moreover, the treatment is expensive. In spite of their hectic lives, Meena's caring aunt and uncle found some time to open up their home and hearts to help her. Meena was fortunate to have such loving relatives; she was indeed born lucky.

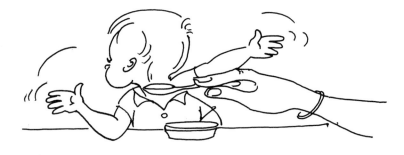

He Knows Best

Mr. and Mrs. Osborn, a very charming couple in their thirties, did not have any children and finally adopted a toddler, whom they named Dennis. I took care of Dennis for the usual childhood diseases and routine immunizations in the outpatient clinic. The Osborns were happy that things were turning out so well. Dennis was quite active and had the usual quota of falls and bruises. As bruises began to appear even for minor injuries, the Osborns became worried and brought him to the hematology clinic. Because he had been adopted, his family history was unknown. Dennis looked normal except for multiple bruises, especially over his legs. There were no enlarged lymph glands. Liver and spleen were not enlarged, either, but a routine blood check showed a very low number of platelets. Platelets play an important role in blood clotting; when they are low, bruising occurs even with minor injuries, as well as bleeding under the skin. Dennis's hemoglobin was also low. However, his white cell count was higher than normal, with an increased number of lymphocytes. A blood smear revealed many immature lymphocytes called "lymphoblasts". This was bad news. A bone marrow test immediately confirmed that Dennis had lymphoblastic leukemia.

The Osborns were devastated. We convinced them that the treatment for leukemia had become more sophisticated and that Dennis had a greater than 50 percent chance of survival (the cure rate today is 80 percent). We started Dennis on medications to lower his high uric acid level; he was also started on chemotherapy. To eliminate residual cancer cells, Dennis was given radiation to his brain. All of this made him sick and he needed a few admissions to the hospital. At the end of the initial treatment, Dennis's bone marrow revealed no lymphoblasts, indicating that he was in remission. Naturally, the Osborns were happy.

Unfortunately, within a few weeks, the leukemia came back with a vengeance. No chemotherapeutic agent could touch Dennis. His platelet counts fell so low that he started to bleed. Repeated platelet and packed cell transfusions alleviated his condition temporarily, and we kept him comfortable with pain-killing medications. Dennis passed away peacefully, four months after the initial diagnosis.

Again, Mr. and Mrs. Osborn were devastated. We sat in a room with a nurse and another physician who had helped in the chemotherapy. Mr. Osborn looked at me, eyes swollen from crying, and asked, "Dr. Rao, tell me, why my son? We didn't have a child and Dennis came into our lives. He was our sunshine. We attend church regularly. Why did the Lord, who gave us Dennis, take him away so early in his life? Why?"

I thought for a moment and replied, "Mr. Osborn, why God takes away someone you love, early, is hard to fathom. With our limited faculties, it is impossible to understand the doings of the Limitless. He loved Dennis. Perhaps, Dennis was needed in another part of the universe, for the betterment of the universe. The Lord knows best."

I held their hands in silence. Sometimes silence conveys feelings better than any words.

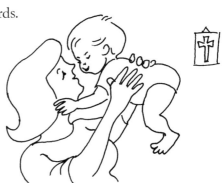

Tornado Phobia

*M*rs. Sandoval brought Richard to my office for a peculiar problem—the eight-year-old was afraid to open any window in the house; and if someone else did, he would scream, jump up and down, get panicky, and sweat profusely. Once the windows were closed he would calm down.

Mrs. Sandoval was at her wit's end. She told me that Richard had recently watched a video of a tornado devastating a town. Cars and trucks flew away, buildings collapsed, and people died. He was now afraid that a tornado would somehow sneak into their house through an open window and devastate their house and family. While talking with me, Mrs. Sandoval realized that Richard's fear of open windows and tornadoes had started after watching the video.

"Could this be the cause of Richard's problem?" she asked.

"It could," I replied.

The average American family leaves the TV set on for seven hours a day; many families keep it on just to provide background noise. Sixty percent of all families have the TV on during meal times. As a result, the average American child spends approximately 28 hours a week in front of the television set, the single biggest chunk of time spent in the waking life of a child. Violent acts appear 8 to 12 times an hour on prime time television, and about 20 times an hour in children's programs that include cartoons. In other words, children watch over 12,000 acts of violence on TV in a year. This is outrageous, particularly because there is a strong correlation between children's exposure to media violence and various behavioral and psychological problems.

"Richard," I said, "I've been in Porterville for twenty-one years. I haven't seen a tornado here, so the chances of your house being struck by a tornado are almost nil."

This fact did not impress Richard.

"Do you believe in God?" I asked.

"Yes," he replied.

"God is very powerful. He can easily control a tornado. Right?"

"Yes"

"So every night, before going to bed, sincerely pray to God to protect you against tornadoes. I assure you that He'll listen to your prayers and help you," I said.

I told Mrs. Sandoval that, in addition to praying, she should leave Richard's bedroom window open a little after a few days. If Richard tolerated it, she should leave the window open a little more every three days or so. I advised her to call me if any panic attacks ensued.

Richard did well. With prayer and incremental opening of the windows, he got over his tornado phobia. I felt happy that Richard's problem was solved without resort to using any medications.

Some movies and television programs are unsuitable for young children. Parents should limit children's TV watching and should censor children from viewing violent and emotional programs. In this respect, it will greatly help if parents themselves could refrain from watching violent programs and thus set an example for their children.

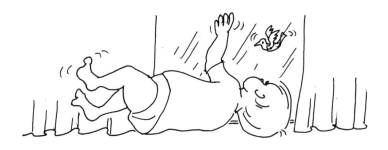

The Benefits of Prayer

*L*inda had a cancer of the lymph glands called non-Hodgkin's lymphoma. After the initial chemotherapy and radiation, the doctors in a children's hospital gave me a treatment road map so I could give her various drugs. Periodically, I put up an IV drip in my office and gave her intravenous medications with weird names such as Vincristine, Cytoxan, and Daunorubicin.

Because of them, Linda stopped eating, became weak, lost her hair, and got depressed. Her mother was devastated. During that time, we talked about prayer. It is well known that praying regularly, especially at times of stress and calamity, will alleviate the consequent sorrow and depression. In fact, in some cancer centers, meditation and prayer are practiced as a routine part of cancer treatment, especially for incurable cancers.

How do prayer and meditation help to improve the well-being of ordinary people and of patients with incurable diseases?

Neurologists, using a technique called PET brain scanning, have studied Buddhist monks during their prayer and deep meditation sessions. They found that, during these sessions, activity in an area over the parietal lobes of the brain slowed down to a remarkable extent. Normally, this area of the brain is very active and orients the human body in physical space, so that one realizes that he or she is different from the surroundings. However, when activity in this area slows down very much, as it occurred in the monks, the distinction between self and surroundings breaks down. At such times, the person becomes one with the universe and has visions of light or of God.

Whether the perception of oneness occurs with nature or with God depends on many factors such as culture, education, faith, prior beliefs, peer groups, and parental practices. Christians envision Christ, and Hindus envision the Lord Krishna, and so on, depending on their religious beliefs. Perhaps mystics see God and angels because of this neurological change in the brain. In patients with cancer and other incurable diseases, the same phenomenon may occur during meditation and prayer, thus decreasing discomfort and pain.

If quieting an area of the brain makes one perceive God or have a similar experience, then, is there really a God or is He an illusion of the brain? I recollect a story wherein a scientist approached God to say there was no longer a need for Him, as scientists could create life by cloning and other methods.

"Let me see how you create life," God said, and smiled.

The scientist picked up some dust and proceeded to produce life.

"Wait a minute," said God, interrupting him.

When the scientist looked up inquiringly, God explained, "I made that dust. If you want to create life, make your own dust first!"

Even if scientists in the future can explain the origins of the universe, there will still remain questions such as what was there before the universe came into being, why and where did it all come from, and so on. Science can go only so far. Beyond that, I believe, it is God's will.

Linda and her mother told me that they felt better after the prayers. Linda recovered fully from cancer after completing several courses of chemotherapy.

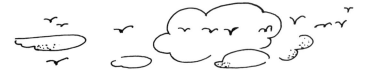

God's Gift

I was called to the newborn nursery to see an infant, Carlos Hernandez, who was described as having "peculiar" facial features.

Mrs. Hernandez was thirty-nine years old and in good health. She denied taking any drugs or alcohol during her pregnancy and there was no history of consanguinity. She did not consent to an amniocentesis or an ultrasound study during her prenatal visits. She had two sisters who were developmentally disabled and wheelchair bound.

Carlos was her tenth child. He was cute, with small "c" shaped ears, slightly slanted eyes, flattened nasal bridge, a small mouth, and a big tongue. All these features gave him a peculiar face. He had a single crease on the right palm and his nails were narrow and convex. His toes overlapped and his muscles were slightly flabby. All these gave me an impression that Carlos had Down syndrome.

Even though this syndrome is named after the British surgeon, John Langdon Down, who described it in detail in 1866, it was actually recognized as early as 1838 by J. E. D. Esquinol. However, its cause was discovered only recently, in 1959. Down syndrome is a chromosomal clinical abnormality. Chromosomes are made up of DNA and other protein complexes and contain most of the genetic information that is passed from parents to children. Instead of forty-six chromosomes, which we normally have, Carlos had forty-seven chromosomes in all the cells of his body. The two chromosomes of his 21st pair were replaced by three, which I found later with chromosomal analysis.

What does this mean? This one extra chromosome creates

multiple problems. Children with Down syndrome have varying degrees of mental retardation. They may have or develop problems with the heart, eyes, ears, spine, thyroid, and the nervous system.

In the past, all children with Down syndrome were looked at differently and most of them were institutionalized, but in the early 1960s President John F. Kennedy established a national commission for mental retardation that introduced sweeping changes.

Now people are aware of the strengths and rights of individuals with disabilities and have come to accept that persons with Down syndrome can be cared for within the home environment. They have better access to medical care and can receive proper attention for their special needs. Consequently, in the absence of seizures and major organ malformations, the mildly retarded child will eventually achieve a sixth grade academic level and be capable of economic independence. The moderately retarded child will be able to be employed in sheltered workshops and to live in group homes. Profoundly retarded children need to be trained in self-help skills. Some may need group home settings; some others may require institutional placement.

Regardless of the predicted long-term capabilities and placement, the optimal environment for the Down syndrome child is with the family.

Burdened with all these thoughts, I entered Mrs. Hernandez's room, briefly explained Carlos' diagnosis, and outlined possible developmental problems. Although I was bringing her bad news, I pointed out that there were still many good things we could do to make Carlos' life comfortable and useful. I told her that we would obtain assistance from the genetics division of the children's hospital, from children's services, and from the regional center.

Mrs. Hernandez listened carefully and said, "Dr. Rao, one of my friends has a child with Down syndrome and I'm familiar with some of the problems. I'm not worried. This is my child; I will raise him as I did my other children. It is God's will that I should have this child, and I consider him a special gift from God."

Four years have gone by. Carlos, with his elder siblings, comes to my office for routine checkups. Children with Down syndrome are cute in their own way and the siblings enjoy Carlos' company. They play with him and teach him to talk. When he imitates them, they all laugh wholeheartedly. Simple acts, such as taking a lollipop from my hand without dropping it, have made the family very proud of Carlos. They consider raising Carlos as a challenge that has given them a special purpose in their lives. In that process, they derive a lot of happiness.

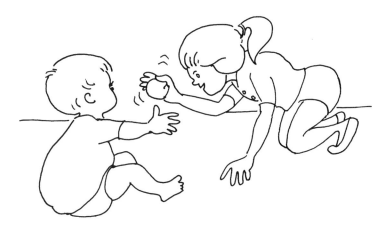

The Lighter Side of My Practice

On my office practice, not a day goes by without a humorous or unique experience tickling me. Children are honest and spontaneous, just like four-year-old Brad. When he came out of my examination room, I offered him a lollipop. Brad's mother looked at him expectantly.

"What do you say to the doctor, Brad?" she asked. She told me that she was teaching Brad his manners and he was learning fast. As Brad simply started to lick the lollipop, his mother again prompted him, "Brad, what do you say to the doctor?"

Brad stopped licking, and looking at me innocently, said, "Can I have one more candy, please?"

Children love to share information; after all, this is the information-sharing age. Children nowadays know much more than we think they do.

"I know a secret!" five-year-old Tara whispered in my ear.

"What is it? Can you please tell me?" I whispered back. Tara's mother, thin and beautiful, was smiling and wondering what the secret was.

"My mom is pregnant!" Tara announced, as her mother's face turned pink with embarrassment.

Some children are very definite about the treatment they want. The other day, Sean came to my office for a physical that he needed before he could enter first grade.

"What can I do for you, Sean?" I asked as I entered the room.

"He knows what he wants. Tell him, Sean," his mother prompted.

"I need a rooster shot!" Sean announced proudly.

Mothers too are sometimes confused about medical

terminology. Mothers have told me that their children were suffering from "ammonia" when they had pneumonia. For minor cuts they have used "neosperm" ointment, when they actually had used neosporin ointment. One mother wanted me to call in a prescription for her son's "E. Coli orgasms" in the urine; actually they were E. Coli organisms. That mother knew a laboratory technician who had informed her about the germs in the urine.

Talking about laboratory personnel, there was a new employee in a lab many years ago. One day, I needed the value of bilirubin in a newborn. Bilirubin is a yellow pigment that is elevated in jaundiced babies. I called the lab employee and said, "I need bilirubin results done today."

"How do you spell it?" asked the employee before I had completed my request.

I spelled it out for him, slowly, "BILI". I paused. "RUBIN."

I was put on hold. After a while, the employee answered, "Dr. Rao, there are no results available on Baby Rubin."

Laughter is the best medicine. When the days are long and the going is rough, humorous events and children's laughter help me to keep my poise. James Barrie said, "When the first baby laughed for the first time, the laugh broke into a thousand pieces and they all went skipping about, and that was the beginning of fairies." Laughter that breaks into a thousand pieces, and goes skipping all around? No doctor's office, and certainly no home, should be without it!

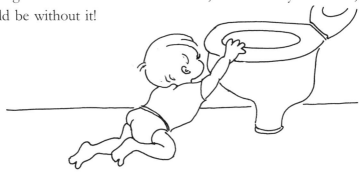

Afterthoughts

One day, Mrs. Morgan said to me, full of gratitude, "Dr. Rao, you've saved my Brenda's life. You're a good doctor, and I thank you."

"Mrs. Morgan, the truth is that Brenda saved herself," I replied. "Of course we all helped." Brenda, the fifteen-year-old who had cancer of her lymph nodes, had suffered the agony of radiation, week after week of chemotherapy, and the humiliation of hair loss. The gnawing pain and constant stress depressed her and she cried, scared that she would not make it. But against all odds, she recovered, fell in love, got married, and gave birth to a girl!

How was Brenda able to cope with such a normally devastating illness? I feel it was because she had a very positive attitude, a firm belief in herself, strong faith in God, and the unflinching support of her family and friends.

"How do you handle stress?" I asked another parent, Mrs. Ramos, who is raising a child with muscular dystrophy. She knows there is no cure for the disease.

"One day at a time," she solemnly replied. "I have read and continue to read everything I can lay my hands on about the disease. I know what will happen to my son, but I don't dwell on it. I get help from relatives and from the community. One day at a time. That's how I handle stress."

Any disease can cause stress, more so those of a chronic nature. Modern technology does not lessen the pain and anguish of a child suffering from cancer, or the anxiety caused by a bully at school; however, you can reduce stress by cultivating a positive attitude, accepting that some events cannot be changed, exercising regularly, eating balanced meals, and getting enough rest and sleep. Relaxation methods, such as meditation, prayer, and special breathing techniques will help to a great extent. Such skills are helping to alleviate the stress and anxiety of cancer patients in the Stress Reduction Clinic at the University of Massachusetts Medical Center.

Above all, make sure you communicate with your doctor and know exactly the ins and outs of your child's disease, medications that have been prescribed, their side effects, and how to cope with them. In addition, take advantage of social services, counseling, support groups, and other community resources.

I pondered over Mrs. Morgan's earlier comment. Who is a good doctor? In my opinion, a pediatrician who communicates well, listens to you and to your child, naturally loves children, is compassionate, has empathy, and puts the healthcare of children before his reimbursements is a good doctor. Of course he should be knowledgeable in his field.

How do you choose a good doctor? Certainly not by flipping

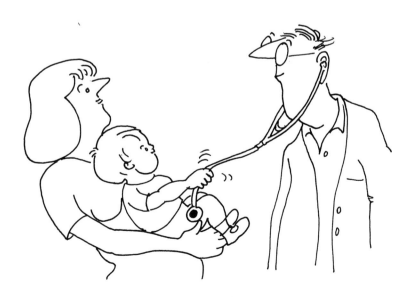

through the yellow pages! Talk to those of your friends who have children and ask them who they take their children to. Why do they like this doctor? Is he or she knowledgeable? How is the office staff? Do they return your calls within a reasonable time? Talk to the receptionist. What are the office hours, and is he or she available after hours and on weekends? Who covers when the doctor is away? Is the doctor board-certified, and does he or she admit patients to a nearby hospital?

All these questions will help you to choose your doctor. You can even call the State Medical Boards to find whether there have been any problems about a particular doctor. It is your child's health that you are concerned about; you don't need to go to a doctor you don't like or do not trust.

Nowadays, raising children has become a challenge because of changing values and ideals, shrinking family size, and constant exposure to a media full of undesirable contents.

In a child's growth and development, the first few years are the most important. Babies are learning machines; they absorb a wealth of information like a sponge. The more they are stimulated, the more they learn. As parents, take every opportunity to interact with your children, physically, intellectually, and emotionally. Simple acts, such as crooning a tune, hugging, playing peek-a-boo, and reading a book aloud will stimulate growth and development in children. But learning is a lifelong process. So, with love, patience, and commitment, make every effort to engage your older children in activities that are conducive to their growth, and to their becoming responsible citizens.

Others in the community beside parents can guide children in their journey to adulthood. The neighborhood, the local church, library, school, doctor, and the local media should also pitch in. These different strata of the community are well suited to educate children and adolescents in several areas, such as sex education, safety rules, health tips, and moral values. Truly, it takes a village to raise a child!

Childhood infections, the "bugs", can be handled with appropriate antibiotics and vaccinations. Children who grow in families with good communication and exemplary role models are less prone to violence and abuse of drugs. Babies who are hugged often and reared with tender loving care grow up confident and optimistic.

Children make up the future. That future entirely depends upon how we raise our children now.

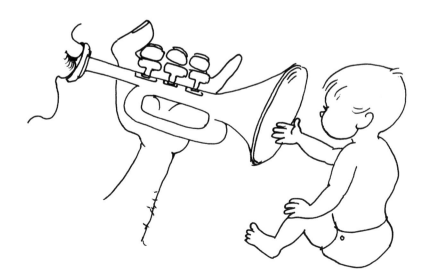

FURTHER READING

1. Benjamin Spock, M.D. and Steven J. Parker, M.D., *Baby and Child Care* (New York: Pocket Books, 1998.)

2. Donald E. Greydanus, M.D., Ed.-in-Chief and Other Editors, *Caring for Your Adolescent, Ages 12 to 21* (New York: Bantam Books, 1994.)

3. Donald Schiff, M.D. and Steven P. Shelov, M.D., *American Academy of Pediatrics Guide to Your Child's Symptoms, The Official, Complete Home Reference, Birth Through Adolescence* (New York: Villard Books, 1997.)

4. Edward L. Schor, M.D., Ed.-in-Chief and Other Editors, *Caring for Your School-Age Child, Ages 5 to 12* (New York: Bantam Books, 1999.)

5. Hillary Rodham Clinton, *It Takes A Village and Other Lessons Children Teach Us.* (New York: Simon & Schuster, 1996.)

6. Jon Kabat-Zinn, Ph.D., *Full Catastrophe Living, Using the Wisdom of Your Body and Mind to Face Stress, Pain, and Illness* (New York: Delta, Dell Publishing, 1991.)

7. Meyer Friedman, M.D and Gerald W. Friedland, M.D., *Medicine's 10 Greatest Discoveries* (New Haven, CT: Yale University Press, 1998.)

8. Randolph M. Nesse, M.D. and George C. Williams, Ph.D., *Why We Get Sick, The New Science of Darwinian Medicine* (New York: Vintage Books, 1996.)

9. Stephen Arterburn & Jim Burns, *Parents Guide to Top 10 Dangers Teens Face* (Wheaton, IL: Tyndale House, 1999.)

10. Steven P. Shelov, M.D., Ed., *Caring for Your Baby and Young Child, Birth to Age 5* (New York: Bantam Books, 1998.)

11. Yosef Geshuri, Ph.D., *Balance of Power in the Family, Behavior Problems with Children: Who is Really in Control at Home* (Porterville, CA: BrainShare Publishing, 2002.)

Index